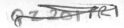

COPING WITH BREAST CANCER

TERRY PRIESTMAN is a consultant clinical oncologist working at New Cross Hospital, Wolverhampton.
He is also medical reviewer for the charity Cancerbackup (which provides infor   for cancer
patients, their relatives and hea   ionals). He
has written more than a hundre   he me ical
press, and is a past Dean o°   of (ical
 ncology at the Royal Col'   gist

Overcoming Common Problems Series

Selected titles
A full list of titles is available from Sheldon Press,
36 Causton Street, London SW1P 4ST, and on our website at
www.sheldonpress.co.uk

Assertiveness: Step by Step
Dr Windy Dryden and Daniel Constantinou

Breaking Free
Carolyn Ainscough and Kay Toon

Calm Down
Paul Hauck

Cataract: What You Need to Know
Mark Watts

Cider Vinegar
Margaret Hills

Comfort for Depression
Janet Horwood

Confidence Works
Gladeana McMahon

Coping Successfully with Pain
Neville Shone

Coping Successfully with Panic Attacks
Shirley Trickett

Coping Successfully with Period Problems
Mary-Claire Mason

Coping Successfully with Prostate Cancer
Dr Tom Smith

Coping Successfully with Ulcerative Colitis
Peter Cartwright

Coping Successfully with Your Hiatus Hernia
Dr Tom Smith

Coping Successfully with Your Irritable Bowel
Rosemary Nicol

Coping with Alopecia
Dr Nigel Hunt and Dr Sue McHale

Coping with Anxiety and Depression
Shirley Trickett

Coping with Blushing
Dr Robert Edelmann

Coping with Bowel Cancer
Dr Tom Smith

Coping with Brain Injury
Maggie Rich

Coping with Candida
Shirley Trickett

Coping with Chemotherapy
Dr Terry Priestman

Coping with Childhood Allergies
Jill Eckersley

Coping with Childhood Asthma
Jill Eckersley

Coping with Chronic Fatigue
Trudie Chalder

Coping with Coeliac Disease
Karen Brody

Coping with Cystitis
Caroline Clayton

Coping with Depression and Elation
Patrick McKeon

Coping with Down's Syndrome
Fiona Marshall

Coping with Dyspraxia
Jill Eckersley

Coping with Eating Disorders and Body Image
Christine Craggs-Hinton

Coping with Eczema
Dr Robert Youngson

Coping with Endometriosis
Jo Mears

Coping with Epilepsy
Fiona Marshall and Dr Pamela Crawford

Coping with Fibroids
Mary-Claire Mason

Coping with Gout
Christine Craggs-Hinton

Coping with Heartburn and Reflux
Dr Tom Smith

Coping with Incontinence
Dr Joan Gomez

Coping with Long-Term Illness
Barbara Baker

Coping with Macular Degeneration
Dr Patricia Gilbert

Coping with the Menopause
Janet Horwood

Overcoming Common Problems Series

Overcoming Common Problems Series

Overcoming Common Problems

Coping with Breast Cancer

Dr Terry Priestman

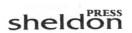
sheldon PRESS

First published in Great Britain in 2006
Sheldon Press
36 Causton Street
London SW1P 4ST

British Library Cataloguing-in-Publication Data
A catalogue for this book is available from the British Library

ISBN-13: 978–0–85969–968–6
ISBN-10: 0–85969–968–4

1 3 5 7 9 10 8 6 4 2

Typeset by Deltatype Limited, Birkenhead, Merseyside
Printed in Great Britain by Ashford Colour Press

To Vera Jackman

Contents

Introduction

Breast cancer is a major health problem worldwide; every year more than a million new cancers will be diagnosed.

In Britain every year about 40,000 women will find they have breast cancer, and overall about one in nine women will develop the condition at some time during their lives. The risk of getting the disease increases with age: half of all breast cancers are first diagnosed in women over the age of 65, and a quarter are first diagnosed in women over the age of 75.

For reasons that nobody fully understands, breast cancer is getting more common. The number of new cases each year in the UK has almost doubled over the last 40 years. Although this increase in the frequency of the disease is worrying, it is offset by the news that the cure rate is rapidly improving. In the early 1990s only about half of all women who had breast cancer could expect to live ten years or more, but now this figure has increased to more than seven out of ten, and is expected to improve further over the coming years. So, most women who get breast cancer can expect to be cured.

The fact that you are likely to survive your breast cancer, and be cured, is great, but being told you have the condition is still a shattering blow for most women, and coming to terms with that diagnosis and living through the months or even years of treatment that might be needed is still anything but easy.

The purpose of this book is to try and help you through that cancer journey. One of the cornerstones of coming to terms with what is happening to you once your cancer has been discovered is information: information about what breast cancer is, how it is treated, and what might happen. One of the two main aims of this book is to give you that information simply and clearly, and to provide the contact details for a number of organizations that can give you more details if you want them. The other aim is to offer some tips and advice on how to cope with living with a diagnosis of breast cancer and getting on with life as normally as possible.

Although breast cancer is the commonest cancer in women today, accounting for one in three of all female cancers, it can also occur in men, although it is very much less common – only about one in 2,000 men will ever get breast cancer during their lifetime. Because it is mainly women who are affected, most of this book has been written with them in mind, but there is a separate chapter on male breast cancer, and much of what is covered in the other chapters applies to men who get the disease.

A final bit of good news is that treatment for breast cancer is improving all the time, with new drugs being discovered and new ways of making better use of existing treatments being developed. This book gives a snapshot of how things are at the end of 2005; one of the frustrations for the author, and benefits for the reader, is that very soon some bits of the information in it will become out of date as beneficial new treatments are introduced – but that is progress.

Terry Priestman
December 2005

1
The big questions

Can it be cured? Will I get better? Will it come back? Am I going to die? How long have I got? Will I be in pain?

When you are first told that you have breast cancer, and have got over the initial shock of the news, these are the sort of questions that are going to be top of your list.

There is some good news.

For many years after records were first kept there was no sign that the results of breast cancer treatment were making any progress, but over the last 15 to 20 years there have been big improvements, and the trend is for things to continue getting better in the future.

In the early 1990s, only about 50 out of every 100 women who had breast cancer could expect to survive ten years or more, and probably be cured. But the latest results show that for every 100 women who first find they have cancer in 2005, more than 70 will be alive in ten years' time. Another way of looking at these figures is that, with 41,000 women being diagnosed with breast cancer each year in the UK, today nearly 8,000 more women every year can expect to live ten years or more, and be cured of their breast cancer, than was the case 15 years ago.

So, being told you have a breast cancer is not a death sentence, and the chances are that you will have a complete cure.

If you are unlucky enough to be one of the minority of women whose breast cancer does come back, there is still some encouragement to offer. Improvements in treatment in recent years mean that even with advanced breast cancer that has spread to other parts of the body, it is still very often possible to live for years – and to be feeling well and enjoying a good quality of life for most of that time.

For many people the word 'cancer' means pain. But pain is not a feature of breast cancer. Certainly for women with early breast cancer, that has not spread, pain is unlikely to be a problem. In fact the main symptoms will come from side-effects of treatment rather than the cancer itself. Although some of these side-effects can be upsetting and a nuisance, such as tiredness or sickness or hot flushes, pain is not part of the picture. With advanced breast cancer, pain can be more of an issue, especially when the cancer has spread to the bones, but usually treatment will be able to get this under complete control and keep any discomfort to a minimum. So although going through treatment for early breast cancer or living with advanced cancer will be tough at times, pain should not be a big problem.

No one is going to welcome the news that they have breast cancer; it is a life-changing event with a huge emotional impact. But the chances are you will come through, and be cured, and be able to pick up the pieces to face the future with confidence and optimism.

2
Why me? What causes breast cancer?

Why me? Why did I get breast cancer? Could I have done anything to stop it? These are very common and understandable questions.

Although we know some factors that make for an increased risk of breast cancer, for many women who get the disease there will really be no obvious cause. We still have a lot to learn about what leads to breast cancer developing. One thing that definitely doesn't cause breast cancer is infection – breast cancer is not something that you can 'catch' from someone else, and it is not caused by a virus or a germ. So even if someone close to you has a breast cancer, there is no way that they can pass it on to you.

Newspapers and magazines are always running stories about possible causes of breast cancer. These are nearly always scientific theories, or unproven ideas, that eventually turn out to be wrong. The two main points that influence a woman's chances of getting breast cancer are her age and her hormones. Another factor that can play a part is breast cancer running in the family, but, although this has received a lot of publicity in recent years, fewer than one in ten cases of breast cancer are actually linked to inheriting faulty genes. Let's look at these, and some of the other points that have been linked to causing breast cancer, in a bit more detail.

Age

Age is the biggest risk factor of all. Overall, one in nine women will get breast cancer in Britain today. But this is what is known as a life-time risk, and the real likelihood of finding a breast cancer increases the older a woman is. Breast cancer before the age of 30 is very, very rare – it can happen but it is extremely unlikely. Between the ages of 30 and 34 one woman in every 50,000 will find she has breast cancer each year, so it is still extremely uncommon. Between 40 and 44 the figure rises to one woman in every 1,000 each year. Ten years later, between the ages of 50 and 54, the risk has increased to one in 500, and by the time you reach the early 80s it is up to one in 250. So, a woman of 81 is about 200 times more likely to find a breast cancer than a woman of 31. In this respect breast cancer is like most other types of cancer, in that the older you are the more likely it is to happen. Quite why this should be no one really knows, but a reasonable explanation is that changes to the cells that make up our bodies are happening all the time, and the longer you live the greater the chance that some of these changes may turn out to be cancerous.

Incidentally, although the risk of breast cancer increases as a woman gets older, the tumours which occur in elderly women are often very slow growing, and usually need less intensive treatment than those that affect younger women.

Hormones: oestrogen

Hormonal factors are very important in breast cancer development. The most important hormone is oestrogen. Oestrogen is the main female hormone. Up to the time of the menopause it is mainly produced in the ovaries, the two walnut-sized organs which sit either side of the womb, deep inside the pelvis. After the menopause, although the ovaries stop producing oestrogen a woman will still make small amounts of the hormone in her adrenal glands (two small organs sitting on top of each of the kidneys) and in the fatty tissues of her body.

Oestrogen levels in the blood are related to the risk of breast cancer developing in several ways. These include:

• The number of years a woman menstruates will affect her risk level: generally speaking, the longer a woman has periods the greater the risk of breast cancer, so starting your periods at a young age, say 10 or 11, and continuing them to a late age, say beyond 50, means you are at a slightly greater risk of breast cancer than a woman who doesn't start her periods till her mid-teens and whose periods have stopped by the age of 45.
• Pregnancy has a protective effect: having children reduces a woman's risk of getting breast cancer, especially if she has her

4

family at a relatively young age. (Incidentally, it has been suggested that having an abortion might increase a woman's likelihood of getting breast cancer, but there is no scientific evidence for this and it is one of the many myths about causes of breast cancer.)

• Breastfeeding also reduces your risk of breast cancer.

So you could argue that the most effective way to reduce a woman's chances of getting breast cancer is to tell her to have as many pregnancies as possible before the age of 20 and breastfeed all her children!

The hormonal factors we have looked at so far are all natural events, but two other situations need to be discussed: hormone replacement therapy (HRT) and taking oral contraceptives.

HRT

HRT has been widely used for many years to help women cope with the more unpleasant symptoms of the menopause. Several recent surveys looking at hundreds of thousands of women who have taken HRT have shown a link to breast cancer, although some of the reports of these results in the media have made this seem more worrying than it really is.

To put things in perspective, first of all there does not appear to be any increase in breast cancer risk for women who take HRT up to the age of 50, so younger women are not affected. Over the age of 50 the degree of risk depends on the type of HRT that has been taken and the length of time it has been taken. There are two main types of HRT; one uses the female hormone oestrogen on its own, the other combines it with the other main female hormone, progesterone. Between the ages of 50 and 64 a total of about 32 women in every 1,000 who have not taken HRT will develop breast cancer. Among women who have taken combined HRT, with oestrogen and progestogen (a man-made form of progesterone), for five years there will be about six more cases of breast cancer, so about 38 in every 1,000; and for women who have taken combined HRT for ten years the figure rises to an extra 19 cases, or about 50 in every 1,000. The risks are lower with oestrogen-only preparation: with this, there would be about one to two extra cases per 1,000 women between the ages of 50 and 64 among those who had taken this type of HRT for five years, and about five extra cases for those women who had taken it for ten years. So although a woman who takes HRT after the age of 50 is increasing her risk of breast cancer, that increase in risk is still quite small, especially if she uses the oestrogen-only tablet and doesn't take it for a long time. Based on these figures we can say:

- Taking HRT up to the age of 50 does not increase the breast cancer risk.
- Over the age of 50 the benefits of using HRT for a short time will outweigh the risks for many women.
- Women over 50 who do take HRT should review this with their family doctor at least once a year.
- Women over 50 who are taking HRT should make sure they attend for regular breast cancer screening.

The pill

As with HRT there are different types of contraceptive pill. The two main ones are combined preparations which include both of the main female hormones, oestrogen and progestogen, and the progestogen-only tablet (sometimes called the mini-pill). There is no evidence linking the progestogen-only mini-pill to breast cancer development; indeed, some experts claim it may even slightly reduce the risk of the condition.

For the combined pill there does seem to be a slight increase in breast cancer risk for younger women who take it for some time: the longer the time, the greater the risk. So, for example, a woman of 25 who takes the combined pill for eight years will have about one and a half times the risk of getting breast cancer compared with a woman who has never taken the pill. But, as we have seen, the chances of getting breast cancer at the age of 33 are very small, about one in 50,000, so this means that the risk has still only increased to about one in 30,000 – very small indeed. Once a woman stops taking the combined pill then her increased risk of breast cancer begins to reduce and has disappeared completely within ten years. Also, the increase in risk seems only to affect younger users of the pill. Women who take the combined pill over the age of 35 do not seem to be any more likely to develop breast cancer than non-users.

Family history and faulty genes

Breast cancer is far and away the commonest cancer in women and so it is not surprising that more than one person may be affected in a family. This does not necessarily mean that there is something that makes members of that family more at risk of developing breast cancer than others. On the other hand, it is well known that some families do carry a higher risk than normal of breast cancer occurring.

Over the years experts have worked out how to tell whether a family does or does not have this greater risk. To do this they look at the numbers and types of cancer within a family. All the cancers have to be on the same side of the family (the mother's side or the father's side) and affect either a first- or second-degree relative. A first-degree relative is a mother, father, daughter, son, sister or brother; a second-degree relative is a grandparent, a grandchild, an aunt, an uncle, a niece, a nephew or a half-sister or half-brother. If a woman has any of the following then she is at more than moderate risk of getting breast cancer at some time during her life:

- one first-degree and one second-degree female relative who had breast cancer diagnosed before the age of 50;
- two first-degree female relatives diagnosed with breast cancer before the age of 50;
- three or more first- or second-degree female relatives diagnosed with breast cancer at any age;
- one first-degree male relative diagnosed with breast cancer at any age;
- one first-degree female relative who has had cancer affecting both breasts (bilateral breast cancer), where the first cancer was discovered before the age of 50;
- one first- or second-degree relative with cancer of the ovary at any age and one first- or second-degree female relative with breast cancer (at least one of these should be a first-degree relative).

7

If a woman has any of these risk factors her family doctor will refer her to specialists to look more closely at her family history and work out the real risks, both for her and for other members of her family. Fewer than one woman in 100 will be at high risk because of her family history. If there does seem to be a high risk then they may go on to do genetic testing. This looks to see if members of the family are carrying a faulty gene which might cause breast cancer.

The genes are the microscopic chemical parcels in our cells which carry all the information that controls how our cells develop and how our bodies grow and behave. We now know that some cancers are caused by faulty genes. For breast cancer two abnormal genes have been discovered: these are called BRCA1 and BRCA2. If a woman has one of these faulty genes in her cells then there is an 85 per cent chance she will get breast cancer some time during her life, which compares with the normal risk of about 12 per cent. However, only a small minority of women with a strong history of breast cancer have been found to have one of these abnormal genes. Even among women who have four or more first- or second-degree relatives with breast cancer, only one in three will have either the BRCA1 or BRCA2 gene.

Just to put the risks in perspective for women who do have a family history of breast cancer but no evidence of the BRCA1 or BRCA2 gene: of 100 'normal' women 12 will develop breast cancer during their lifetime; of 100 women who have had a first-degree relative with breast cancer the figure rises to about 17; and with two first-degree relatives affected it would be about 25, or more or less double the normal risk.

Race

Does your ethnic background make a difference to your chances of getting breast cancer? The answer is: yes, there are some variations.

If you are a black African or Caribbean woman, your risk of getting breast cancer is about the same as Caucasian (white) women living in the UK. But if you come from a southern Asian family, from Bangladesh, India or Pakistan, then you are rather less at risk: about one in 14 south Asian women get breast cancer compared to about one in nine in the general female population. If your racial background is from the Far East, China or Japan, for example, then your risk is even lower and is only about half that of the general population.

So for every 100 white or black African-Caribbean women, about 14 will get breast cancer at some time during their lives, for south Asian women this number falls to about 11, and for women from the Far East it is lower still, with about seven out of every 100 women being at risk.

Lifestyle

There is a huge amount of misinformation produced about the links between diet and breast cancer. In fact, although countless studies have been done, there is actually no good scientific evidence linking food with either an increased or reduced risk of breast cancer. There is a popular belief that a diet rich in dairy products (milk, butter and cheese) makes breast cancer more likely, but although scientists have looked at this very carefully there does not appear to be any link between the two. Similarly, there is no strong evidence to suggest that eating a lot of red meat puts a woman at risk of breast cancer (although there may well be a link with bowel cancer). By the same token, there is no evidence that vegetarians, or people who eat a diet rich in fruit and vegetables, are less likely to develop breast cancer (although eating plenty of fruit and vegetables is very good from a general health point of view).

The only definite link between what you eat and drink and breast cancer is alcohol. Women who drink regularly are more at risk of getting breast cancer, and the more alcohol they drink the greater that risk becomes. So drinking a glass of wine every day would increase a woman's chances of getting breast cancer by about 5 per cent, or one in 20; drinking two glasses of wine every day would increase the risk by about 10 per cent, or one in ten, and so on.

Incidentally, a few years ago there were a number of stories suggesting that drinking a lot of coffee could lead to breast cancer. This is another myth. Although drinking a great deal of coffee, with lots of caffeine, may not be good for you for other reasons, there is no reliable evidence to show that it causes breast cancer.

Related to diet is the question of weight, and here again there is some clear evidence. Women who are past their menopause and who are overweight are more at risk, possibly because their extra fatty tissue leads to an increase in oestrogen production in their bodies. Women over the age of 50 who are actually obese are about twice as likely to get breast cancer as women of normal weight.

Linked to excess weight is the question of exercise. Here studies have shown a clear benefit from regular exercise. Even modest exercise, say walking about half an hour every day, definitely reduces a woman's chance of getting breast cancer.

Perhaps surprisingly, although it is the major cause of lung cancer and increases the risk of many other types of cancer, there is no link between cigarette smoking and breast cancer. But, because of its many other health risks like heart disease, circulatory problems and strokes, smoking is definitely not a good idea, and there is certainly no suggestion that it actually reduces the risk of breast cancer.

Another lifestyle factor where there is a lot of misunderstanding is stress. Newspaper and magazine articles regularly report that stress can lead to breast cancer. This is completely untrue. Many studies have looked at this question and almost all show no link at all – in fact, there is even the suggestion that women who experience a lot of stress are actually less likely to get breast cancer.

Hair dyes and antiperspirants (underarm deodorants) are also sometimes claimed to be linked to breast cancer but once again there is no good scientific evidence for this.

Can you prevent breast cancer?

There will be a small minority of women where a very strong family history, with or without the presence of one of the abnormal breast cancer genes, will mean they are at a particularly high risk of developing the disease. Depending on their degree of risk their specialists may suggest extra precautions for them. This may simply involve having regular check-ups, to try and ensure that if a cancer does develop it is detected as soon as possible, or they may recommend treatments to try and stop cancers occurring in the first place. These treatments may involve either drugs (chemoprevention) or surgery.

Chemoprevention has been based round the hormonal drug tamoxifen. Clinical trials looking at giving tamoxifen to women at high risk of getting breast cancer have given mixed results, some showing that it may help but others showing no real benefit, so how much it really reduces risk remains an open question. Another drug that is being looked at in this situation is called raloxifene, but at the moment this is still being assessed in clinical trials and it is not clear how effective it will be. Incidentally, there has been a lot of publicity recently about another group of hormonal drugs, called aromatase inhibitors, that may be better than tamoxifen. The aromatase inhibitors include anastrazole (Arimidex), letrozole (Femara) and exemestane (Aromasin). Although these drugs do look to be very effective they only work in women who have passed the menopause, and this limits their usefulness in the role of chemoprevention.

The surgical approach involves an operation to remove both breasts, bilateral mastectomy. This sounds a rather drastic form of prevention but it is very effective, and the studies that have been done show that those women who have looked at their risks and feel they really want this option cope remarkably well with the surgery and the resulting change in their body image. Incidentally, when these precautionary bilateral mastectomies are done it is usual to offer breast reconstruction at the same time, which does help to reduce the cosmetic change from the operation.

For the great majority of women, however, chemoprevention or bilateral mastectomy would not be justified. For those women who want to keep their risk to a minimum then there are some tips:

- If you are over 50, avoid taking HRT other than for a short time.
- If you are over 50, avoid getting overweight.
- Take regular steady exercise.
- Keep your alcohol intake down.

3
What is breast cancer?

A cancer happens when the growth of cells in a part of our body goes wrong.

We are made up of countless millions of cells. We all start from a single fertilized cell in our mother's womb. That cell divides into two, those two cells divide into four, those four cells divide into eight, and so on. In the early weeks of life, as more cells are formed, they begin to change into all the different types that are needed to make our bodies: blood cells, nerve cells, bone cells, muscle cells and many others.

Even when we are adults, and no longer growing, we still go on making millions of new cells every day to replace old cells that have worn out and died off. Our bodies have very precise controls to make sure that the number of new cells produced exactly balances the number of old cells that have been lost, so that everything is kept in balance.

A cancer happens when these controls break down and cells begin to divide and reproduce in an uncontrolled way, making far too many new cells. With time, probably over a number of years, these cells will build up to form a lump – the primary cancer. As this lump gets bigger it will begin to invade the normal tissues around it, eating into and destroying them. Eventually, if this primary cancer has not been discovered and treated, it will send off seedlings of cancer cells into the bloodstream or the lymph vessels, which will be carried to other parts of the body where they will settle and form secondary cancers, or metastases.

Cancer is not a single disease. There are more than 200 different types of cancer. These different cancers are usually named after the part of the body in which the primary cancer first develops. More than half of all the cancers that occur are made up of just four types: breast cancer, bowel cancer, lung cancer and prostate cancer.

What is breast cancer?

Breast cancer is the result of a failure of the controls of normal cell growth, which leads to a primary cancerous lump developing in the breast.

The female breast is designed for producing milk for a newborn baby. It is made up of lots of glands, called lobules, which are turned on at the end of pregnancy to make the breast milk. These lobules drain into fine tubes, called ducts, and the ducts carry the milk to the nipple. The lobules and the ducts are embedded in a mix of fatty and fibrous supporting tissue that makes up the rest of the breast. The structure of the male breast is the same as the female breast, but the lobules and ducts are not so well developed and there is much less fatty and fibrous tissue.

Breast cancers develop from the cells that form the lining of the ducts, or lobules. Usually it is the cells lining the ducts that are the starting point for the disease.

The cells that make the lining, the inner surfaces, of the various organs of our bodies are called epithelial cells. Cancers that are made up of epithelial cells are called carcinomas. So breast cancers are carcinomas of the breast.

At first the cancer cells are confined to the inner lining of either the ducts or the lobules, This earliest stage of the disease is called ductal carcinoma in-situ (DCIS) or lobular carcinoma in-situ (LCIS).

The next stage is when the cancer cells begin to eat into, and invade, the surrounding breast tissue. The tumour has now become an invasive breast cancer. It is also known as the primary breast cancer, because it is the beginning of the disease in the breast. With time the primary breast cancer will grow. The speed of growth varies enormously with different breast cancers; some will get bigger rapidly, over a period of months, whilst, at the other extreme, others will enlarge only slowly, over a period of years.

As the cluster of abnormal, cancerous lining cells begins to grow, it forms a lump. In time this swelling will break through the wall of the duct, or lobule, and begin to invade the surrounding fatty and fibrous tissue in the breast. With time, if this primary cancer has not been removed, it will send off seedlings of secondary cancer.

Usually the first place these secondary cancers go to is into the lymph vessels, which carry them to the lymph nodes under the arm (the axillary lymph nodes) on the same side as the breast – so a cancer in the left breast will spread to the lymph nodes in the left axilla (armpit), and a cancer in the right breast will spread to the right axilla. Later cells will also creep into the blood vessels in the breast and be carried to more distant parts of the body like the bones, the liver, the lungs and the brain.

These secondary cancers in the lymph nodes, or other organs in the body, will be made up of breast cancer cells, and they will be different from the primary cancers that can occur in those sites. So, for example, a secondary breast cancer in the bone will behave completely differently, and need different treatment, from a primary bone cancer. In the same way, a secondary cancer in the liver will still be made up of breast cancer cells and will behave like a breast cancer, not a liver cancer.

Different breast cancers grow at different rates: some very slowly, others much more rapidly. So it is impossible to say how long a breast cancer takes to develop. When people first discover a cancerous lump in their breast a very common question is: how long has it been there? Since the very first cancerous change will have started in a single cell, or a tiny number of cells, within the breast, and since those cells probably multiply only every few weeks or months, it is likely that most breast cancers will have been there for some years before they get big enough to make a lump that can actually be felt, or seen on a breast X-ray (a mammogram). So a breast cancer doesn't develop overnight. Even a very tiny breast cancer, about 0.5cm across, which is about the smallest size that can be detected on X-rays or in the clinic, will contain more than 100 million cancer cells, and will have taken a long time to have grown to that size from that first handful of cancerous cells that started the whole process.

Staging

When doctors are deciding how to treat a breast cancer it is very important for them to know how big it is, whether it has begun to invade into the surrounding breast tissue, whether it has spread, and if it has spread how far it has gone. Finding out this information tells your breast specialists the 'stage' of your cancer, and knowing that stage is very important because different treatments are needed for different stages of the disease.

The earliest stage of a breast cancer is when the cancer cells are only in the lining tissues of the ducts, or lobules, and haven't begun to invade the surrounding breast tissue. This is known as a pre-invasive breast cancer, or carcinoma in-situ. If the growth is in the ducts (which is by far the most common site) it is often called DCIS, the initials standing for ductal carcinoma in-situ; if it is in the lobules then it is LCIS, lobular carcinoma in-situ. These carcinomas in-situ used to be very rare, but since the introduction of breast screening, which can pick up cancers at a much earlier stage in their development, they have become much commoner. About one in five of the cancers discovered at breast screening are pre-invasive in-situ carcinomas.

Over the years doctors have worked out different ways of describing the stages of breast cancer. These staging 'systems' range from the very simple to the very complex. At the simple end of the spectrum, breast cancer can be divided into two stages, early or advanced, 'early' being when the cancer is confined to the breast or has spread only to the axillary lymph nodes, 'advanced' being when it has spread more widely. A slightly more detailed classification divides the life history of breast cancer into four stages:

I The cancer is confined to the breast, and has not invaded either the skin overlying the breast or the muscle beneath it.

II The cancer has involved the axillary lymph nodes.

III The cancer has invaded either the skin of the breast or the muscle underlying it, or both.

IV The cancer has spread beyond the axillary lymph nodes.

The most complicated, but many doctors would say the best, staging system is called the TNM classification. 'T' describes the size of the primary tumour: a Tis lump is an in-situ, pre-invasive cancer, and the invasive cancers are described as T1 to T4 depending on their size and whether or not they have invaded skin or muscle. 'N' describes the spread to the axillary lymph nodes; N0 means there is no spread, N1 to N3 means that there are varying numbers of lymph nodes involved. 'M' refers to more distant spread; if this has happened and there are secondary cancers elsewhere in the body then the stage is M1, if not then it is M0. So, for example, a primary invasive cancer measuring 2cm across, which had spread to involve three lymph nodes under the arm but showed no signs of spread elsewhere, would be a T2N1M0 cancer.

Grading

Another thing that it is important for doctors to know when they come to make treatment decisions is the grade of the cancer.

Grading looks at the appearance of the cancer cells under the microscope. In some cases the cancers will look very similar to normal breast tissue, with only slight changes showing that it really is a cancer. In other cases the cells will look very abnormal indeed and have little in common with normal breast tissue. Sometimes the appearances are in between these two extremes.

When the cancer looks very like normal tissue it is called 'well differentiated', or a Grade I cancer. When it is very abnormal it is called 'poorly differentiated', or a Grade III cancer. When the appearances are in between then that is a 'moderately differentiated' or a Grade II cancer.

Usually, but not always, the grade predicts how that cancer will behave, with Grade III cancers being more aggressive, more rapidly growing and more likely to spread than Grade II cancers, and Grade I cancers being the slowest growing and least likely to spread.

Hormone receptors

Sex hormones are the chemicals our bodies make which control many of the aspects of our appearance and behaviour. In men the sex hormones are called androgens, and the most important of these is testosterone. In women the main sex hormone is oestrogen, and they also produce a hormone called progesterone.

Up to the time of the menopause oestrogen and progesterone are made by the ovaries, the two small, walnut-sized glands that lie either side of the womb, deep in the pelvis. After the menopause oestrogen production continues, although at a much lower level, with the hormone being made in the adrenal glands (two small glands which sit on top of each of the kidneys), and also in cells in the fatty tissues of the body.

Many breast cancers rely on oestrogen to support their growth.

The link between oestrogen and breast cancer was first shown by a Glasgow surgeon, George Beatson, at the end of the nineteenth century. He did a series of operations on young women with breast cancer where he removed their ovaries (an oophorectomy), and found that after the surgery the cancers often became smaller, and sometimes even disappeared for a while. Although Beatson's work led to a number of types of hormone treatment for breast cancer it was more than fifty years before scientists found out how the oestrogen worked to nourish the cancer.

What they discovered were oestrogen receptors. These are proteins in the cell which mop up oestrogen which is circulating in the bloodstream. Once that oestrogen has bound to the receptor, the receptor is switched on, or stimulated, and sends signals to the nucleus of the cell which tell it to start the process of cell division. So by turning on the receptor, the oestrogen causes the cell to divide, and the cancer to grow.

We now know that almost two out of every three breast cancers have oestrogen receptors. The older a woman is when her breast cancer is discovered, the more likely it is that receptors will be present. So in women under the age of 40 with breast cancer fewer than half will have oestrogen receptors in their tumours, whereas in women over 70 more than three-quarters will have the receptors.

If a breast cancer has oestrogen receptors it is said to be oestrogen receptor positive, or ER+ (the E comes from the American spelling, 'estrogen'). If there are no oestrogen receptors then the cancer is oestrogen receptor negative, or ER–.

Many breast cancers also have receptors for the other female hormone, progesterone, but this seems less important from a treatment point of view. Tumours with progesterone receptors are called progesterone receptor positive, or PgR+.

Nowadays when a woman has a breast cancer removed it will always be tested to see whether or not it is ER+. This helps on deciding the treatment that might be needed: ER+ cancers are very likely to respond to hormone treatments, but ER– cancers are very unlikely to respond. This means doctors will know in advance whether hormone treatment will or will not help, whereas before the discovery of oestrogen receptors and the development of ER testing it was all a matter of trial and error.

Some breast cancer experts believe tumours that are ER+ carry a better outlook than those that are ER–, but this is still not certain, and many other experts don't feel it makes a great deal of difference to the chances of cure whether the cancer is ER+ or ER–.

HER2 receptors

Although most breast cancers contain oestrogen receptors, many do not. Until recently the compounds that encouraged the growth of these tumours remained a mystery. That mystery has been explained to some extent by the discovery of a group of proteins called human epidermal growth factors – HER for short.

So far, four human epidermal growth factors have been identified: HER1, HER2, HER3 and HER4. We all make these proteins and they circulate in our bloodstreams and help to control the process of normal cell growth. They do this by binding to receptors, special proteins on the surface of the cells. Once the growth factors bind to the receptor, that receptor is stimulated and sends signals to the nucleus of the cell telling it to divide – a very similar process to oestrogen stimulating the oestrogen receptors.

About one in five breast cancers has been found to have much higher levels of receptors for HER2 than normal. This means that these cancers are extra-sensitive to HER2, and this drives their growth and development.

Tests have now been invented that can measure the level of HER2 receptors in breast cancer tissue. Those levels are graded:

- 0–1+ means that a normal amount of the HER2 receptor is present.
- 2+ means that a moderately increased amount of the HER2 receptor is present.
- 3+ means that there is a much higher than normal level of the HER2 receptor.

If tissue from a particular breast cancer has a 3+ level of HER2 then it is said to be HER2 positive (HER2+), which means that the level of HER2 receptors is abnormally high and likely to be a major factor in that cancer's growth.

Research has shown that if a breast cancer is HER2+ it is unlikely to be ER+. In other words, if a cancer has receptors that make it sensitive to oestrogen and hormonal treatments, it is unlikely to have an excess of HER2 receptors, and vice versa. Studies have also suggested that cancers which are HER2+ behave more aggressively, growing more rapidly and being more likely to spread to other parts of the body.

Very importantly, during the 1990s a drug was developed that could interfere with the HER2 receptors. This drug is called trastuzumab (Herceptin). It is a type of drug called a monoclonal antibody, which means it is different from both normal chemotherapy (cytotoxic) drugs and hormone therapies. Trastuzumab works by binding to the receptor and stopping the HER2 growth factor from reaching it and stimulating it.

Trastuzumab is an effective part of the treatment of HER2+ breast cancers. But just as hormone therapies are ineffective in cancers that are ER–, so trastuzumab has no benefit in cancers that are HER2–.

ER and HER2 testing

Testing for oestrogen and HER2 receptors is quite simple and relatively inexpensive.

It is now routine practice in the UK that all new breast cancers will be tested for oestrogen receptors. The test can be done on a very small amount of tumour tissue, and is usually carried out when a biopsy of the cancer is taken in the breast clinic. If it is not done at this time then it will be done when surgery is carried out to remove the breast cancer. So you will always know whether your breast cancer is ER+ or not.

The situation with HER2 testing is changing. Until recently it has only been done for those women who it was felt might have a cancer that was HER2 positive, but the realization that trastuzumab can often be an effective treatment for these cancers has led to more widespread testing, and things are moving to a more universal use of HER2 testing when a breast cancer is first discovered.

Usually the ER and HER2 status of a cancer, whether the receptors are there or not, does not change with time. Also, if a breast cancer spreads, the secondary cancers, or metastases, will usually have the same receptors as the primary tumour from which they came. This means that if you had a breast cancer treated some years ago, and it comes back with secondaries in another part of the body, those secondaries will usually have the same pattern of receptors as your original tumour.

It is also the case that most pathology laboratories keep samples of patients' breast cancers for many years, and these samples can be used to test for receptors. This means that if, say, you had a breast cancer treated three or four years ago which was not tested for HER2 receptors and that cancer has now come back, the pathologists can look at your original cancer cells and test them to see whether or not your primary cancer was HER2+.

4

Breast screening

The earlier a breast cancer is discovered, the more likely it is to be completely cured. This simple fact is the basic truth that is behind the idea of screening for breast cancer.

If a cancer can be found before it has spread outside the breast, or at an even earlier stage when it has not even begun to invade into the tissues within the breast (carcinoma in-situ or pre-invasive cancer), then having a simple operation to take the lump away will almost always lead to a cure. The longer things are left, the more likely the cancer is to spread, and the chance of a cure begins to fade.

How is it done?

The test that is at the heart of breast cancer screening is mammography. This uses a special machine to take X-ray pictures of the breast. These pictures will often show a breast cancer long before it would be possible to feel it as an actual lump in your breast. The test is very simple and only takes a few minutes. It doesn't need any special preparation, you can eat and drink normally before and after the test, and you don't have to take any medicines or tablets to help make it work. The examination may be done at your local hospital or in a mobile breast screening unit which will visit a place near to where you live.

The test is done by specially trained radiographers who will explain everything to you and answer any questions you may have about it. You will have to have your top half undressed, and either stand by, or lie beside, the mammography machine. The radiographers will then take X-ray pictures of each of your breasts in turn, and will take the pictures from two different positions. To get the best pictures the breast often has to be slightly squeezed by the machine; this may be a little bit uncomfortable, and very

22

occasionally some women find it quite painful for a moment or two. Actually taking the pictures is completely painless – you don't feel anything from the X-rays, and the test does not make you radioactive. Afterwards your breasts may feel a little bit tender for a short time, but you should not feel unwell in any way and will be perfectly all right to carry on life as normal immediately afterwards. So, for example, it would be fine for you to drive yourself to and from the test appointment.

Once the X-rays have been taken, the mammogram films will be developed and sent to be examined. This will usually be done by two experts, at least one of whom will be a radiologist, a doctor who specializes in looking at X-rays. National targets mean you should get a letter giving you the result of the test within three weeks. If it is all clear then this is obviously good news. If the experts have found anything that they are worried about then they will either arrange some further tests or make an appointment for you at your nearest hospital with a specialist breast clinic.

Who can have it?

The national breast screening programme in the UK was introduced in the late 1980s. At the present time, under the scheme, women between the ages of 50 and 70 will be invited to take part. There has been a lot of discussion about whether younger women should also be included. At the moment there are two main reasons why this hasn't happened. The first is that, although younger women do get breast cancer, it is much less common in this age group: every year fewer than one woman in every 1,000 between the ages of 40 and 50 will discover a breast cancer, whereas in women between the ages of 50 and 70 the figure rises to more than one in 400. So in the younger age group the chances of discovering a cancer by screening are much lower. Second, in younger women mammograms are less reliable and may well miss cancers. This is because younger women have denser, firmer breasts than older women and the mammograms are not able to get such a clear picture of the tissues within the breast, so a cancer could still be there but not show up on the films.

The reason for having an upper age limit for routine screening is not because breast cancer is no longer likely in the over 70s – in fact, it is very common – but because at that age the cancers usually grow very slowly, and so finding them early is not so important as in younger women. But for those women who are concerned and would like to continue having regular screening, then that choice is open to them.

How often should you have screening?

'Regular' is a very important word in breast cancer screening. Having had a normal mammogram once does not mean that you cannot get breast cancer at some time in the future. So the screening is not a 'one-off': it must be repeated every so often to make sure that everything is still all clear. There has been a lot of debate over the years as to what the best timing is for repeat mammograms, and at the present time the UK system has decided on repeating the test every three years.

This means that within a few months of a woman reaching 50 she should receive an invitation in the post to attend for a mammogram, and thereafter should continue to receive those invitations every three years until she is 70. After that it is up to her whether she would like to carry on having the test or not.

Incidentally, another thing to mention is that having a normal mammogram does not mean that you cannot get cancer anywhere else in your body. The mammogram only checks the breasts, it does not look at other places. And so it is important to still attend for other things, like cervical screening, and to still check out any abnormal symptoms that you may get with your GP.

Are there any problems?

Although mammograms are a very good way of finding early breast cancers they are not perfect. Like all medical tests, they cannot be guaranteed to give the right answer every single time. Overall, in women between the ages of 50 and 70, mammograms will pick up about nine out of every ten cancers. Although this is a good figure, it still means that every so often a woman will have a screening mammogram that seems to be completely normal when in fact she does have a cancer. The other side of this coin is that sometimes a mammogram will suggest that there is a cancer in the breast, and further tests will show that either there was nothing, or the lump was completely benign, non-cancerous. About one in every 20 mammograms that appear to show a cancer will turn out to be false-positives, and unfortunately this can cause some unnecessary anxiety.

Because mammograms do not offer a complete guarantee that all is well, it is still important to be 'breast aware' and periodically check your breasts so that if you do find anything different, or abnormal, you can get it checked up on by your GP. For every 1,000 women in the screening age group who have a normal mammogram, two or three will develop a breast cancer before their next screening appointment (these are known as interval cancers).

And, of course, do attend regularly for the repeat examinations every three years.

Some women worry about the fact that a mammogram is a type of X ray, and this means that they will be exposed to radiation which could itself cause cancer. The dose of radiation with a mammogram is very small, but even so it is true that, statistically speaking, there is a very tiny increase in cancer risk as a result of repeated examinations (the estimate is that for every 100,000 mammograms carried out one new cancer may be caused). However, given the number of cancers discovered, and lives saved, by mammograms, the benefits outweigh the risks by many, many times.

Younger women: other types of screening

Although breast screening for the under 50s is not routine in the UK at the present time there is a small group of younger women for whom some kind of screening might be needed. These are women who have been found to be at very high risk of developing breast cancer, usually because they have a very strong history of breast cancer in their family or have been found to be carrying one of the abnormal breast-cancer causing genes, BRCA1 or BRCA2. Since mammography is much less reliable in these younger women there are two other types of screening test that may be used.

The first of these is breast ultrasound. In this test some jelly is smeared over the skin of the breasts and then a special microphone is gently rubbed over the skin. This takes sound pictures of the breast tissue which will often show up any solid lumps within the breast. The test is done as an out-patient: it only takes a few minutes, it is absolutely painless, and it does not make you feel unwell in way.

The second test is called a magnetic resonance imaging or MRI scan. The test involves lying in a special type of scanner which uses high energy magnetic waves to take pictures of the breast tissue. Although the test is painless it does mean lying in quite an enclosed space for anything up to 45 minutes, which can be upsetting for people who feel claustrophobic. It is also quite noisy.

Breast ultrasound is a very simple, widely available test, and is often used alongside mammograms to help in diagnosing breast cancers. MRI scans are much more specialized and only available at some hospitals; although they can be used to help in detecting breast cancers, they are not a routine test and will only be done under special circumstances.

Some facts and figures

Some figures may help to put breast screening in perspective. In the year 2003–4, 1.4 million women in England had breast screening. This led to 11,000 breast cancers being discovered. About half of these cancers were too small to be felt as lumps in the breast, so they would never have been discovered so early had it not been for the breast screening mammograms. Each year more women are attending for breast screening, and more early, curable cancers are being discovered. The present predictions are that by the year 2010 breast screening will save 1,250 women's lives every year in the UK.

Despite these encouraging results still only about three out of four women who are invited will actually attend for screening, and undoubtedly more lives could be saved if this figure could be increased. One worrying statistic is that women from ethnic minority communities seem less likely to take up the offer of screening, and a lot of work is being done to see how they can be persuaded to take a more active part in the programme.

Although these figures are very encouraging, breast screening is expensive. In England alone the service costs more than £50 million a year, and this cost, together with the fact that mammography is not absolutely reliable and will still give occasional false-negative or false-positive results, does from time to time lead various experts to question how cost-effective breast screening is and whether it should continue. But most people still strongly believe that a service that can offer large numbers of women the chance of a complete cure of their breast cancer is very well worthwhile.

Certainly the advice of this book is that if you are approaching, or within, the breast screening age group of 50 to 70, then you should definitely take advantage of the scheme and be attending for your regular mammograms.

5
How do you know if you've got breast cancer?

What are the signs? What do you look out for? Although many women these days have their cancers discovered by routine breast screening, without having been aware beforehand of any problem with their breasts, the commonest sign of the disease is finding a lump in your breast. Other, less common, signs are a change in the appearance of your breast. This might be dimpling or puckering of the skin in one part of the breast, or changes to the nipple with dry, cracking, peeling skin, like eczema, or there may be bleeding from the nipple. The nipple may also become indrawn or inverted, dipping into the breast instead of sticking out from its surface.

Breast lumps are very common and most will be completely benign, due to cysts or other non-cancerous conditions affecting the breast. But the fact that only about one in ten breast lumps actually turn out to be a cancer does not mean that they should be ignored – no woman should ever have an unexplained lump in her breast. If you discover a lump in your breast you should always see your family doctor to get it checked out.

Having said this, many women have naturally lumpy breasts, and the feel of your breasts, the degree of lumpiness, often changes at different times during your menstrual cycle. Your breasts may also be more tender and sensitive around the time of your periods, but once again this is quite normal. The breasts also feel different at different times of life: they are much firmer and denser in young women, becoming much softer and looser after the menopause. If your breast is naturally lumpy then the lumps are likely to be spread throughout your breast, and to be quite soft and rather vague in their shape and outline, whereas abnormal breast lumps tend to be firmer and more definite in their shape and outline, feeling different to the rest of the surrounding breast tissue.

Breast awareness

Because of the natural changes that occur at different times of the month and with the passage of time, it is important to get to know the normal feel of your breasts: to be breast aware. The way to do this is to regularly look at, and feel, your breasts two or three times each month. Try and get into a routine of doing this, possibly when you come out of the shower, or when you are getting undressed at bedtime. Look at your breasts in the mirror, checking their size and shape, the smoothness of the skin and the prominence, colour and texture of your nipples. Then use the flat of your hand to gently rub and squeeze your breasts, checking their feel, their texture, whether they feel smooth or granular or lumpy. Avoid using the tips of your fingers, prodding or pinching your breasts, as this tends to make the breast tissue feel more lumpy than it really is and to make it seem as though there are lumps there when there aren't any. Do make sure you feel all parts of your breast, and also feel under your arms to make sure there are no swellings there.

By doing this over the months and years you will get to be familiar with how your breasts are, their shape, their texture, the way they change at various times of the month, so that if ever a problem does develop you will be able recognize that something is different, that something has changed out of the ordinary, that the normal pattern has altered, and that you need to get your doctor's advice as to whether or not something is really wrong.

The sort of changes to look out for

These include:

- finding a new, separate, discrete, firm lump in your breast that feels different from the rest of your breast;
- a change in the shape of your nipple, especially if it has become drawn in (inverted);
- a rash on or around one of your nipples;
- any discharge or bleeding from one of your nipples;

- a change in the shape of your breast, with dimpling or puckering of the skin over one part of it;
- a swelling in your armpit;
- a noticeable change in the size of one breast compared to the other.

Being breast aware is important. Along with breast screening for women between the ages of 50 and 70, it is a major way of picking up cancer at an early stage, when it will be most curable. The charity Breast Cancer Care has a free leaflet about breast awareness (freephone 0808 800 6000), or go online at <http://www.breastcancercare.org.uk>. There is more information on the Department of Health website at <http://www.cancerscreening.org.uk/breastscreening/breastawareness.html>.

What do you do if you find a change?

Breast lumps can occur at any age from puberty onwards. In women under the age of 30 breast cancer is very rare; finding a lump at this age means it is almost certainly benign, but even so you should still make a visit to your doctor just to be on the safe side.

Perhaps surprisingly, breast cancers are usually completely painless, so finding a lump that does not cause any pain or discomfort does not mean that it can't be a cancer. Unfortunately quite a few women don't realize this and will ignore a lump in their breast because it is painless, believing that if it doesn't hurt it can't be anything serious. If anything the opposite is true: if a breast lump is painful it is more likely to be benign than malignant, but even so it should still be looked at by your doctor.

What will your family doctor do?

So if you think you have found something different about one of your breasts, a lump or a change in its appearance, and you go to see your family doctor, what will happen?

First he or she will ask you about your problem, what you have found, when you first noticed anything wrong, and whether things are changing. Your doctor will ask about your family medical history, to find out if any of your close relatives have had breast cancer. Your doctor will also probably check a few other details about your general health and make a note of any tablets or medicines that you are taking. He or she will then examine your breasts, maybe also feeling under your arms to check for any enlarged lymph nodes. Once this has been done, your doctor will have to make a decision as to whether to refer you to the breast clinic at your local hospital for a specialist opinion and further tests, or whether it is simply a case of reassuring you and keeping an eye on things at the surgery. In order to help GPs to decide whether or not someone should be referred to hospital, the Department of Health and the National Institute for Clinical Excellence (NICE) have issued guidelines about this to all family doctors. The guidelines say that a woman should be urgently referred if they find any of the following:

- a separate, distinct, hard lump within the breast that has become fixed (this means it cannot be moved between the fingers without pulling on either the muscle tissue behind the breast or the skin overlying the breast);
- in women over the age of 30: a separate, distinct lump which is still present after their next period, or has appeared at some time after they have been through the menopause;
- in women under the age of 30: a discrete lump that is growing in size, or is linked to a family history of breast cancer;
- a woman of any age who has had breast cancer in the past, and finds a new lump;
- an eczema-like rash on one nipple, or the surrounding skin;
- a recent change in the shape of one of the nipples;
- bleeding or blood-stained discharge from one of the nipples.

The guidelines also cover men, and say that if a GP finds a firm lump in one breast in a man aged over 50 then they should also be urgently referred to a specialist breast clinic.

An urgent referral means that you should be seen in the breast clinic within two weeks of having seen your GP.

The guidelines also suggest that a non-urgent, routine referral should be made to the clinic if they find either of the following:

- a new lump in someone under the age of 30, which does not appear to be obviously cancerous, and where there is no clear family history of breast cancer (these lumps will almost certainly prove to be benign, but a check-up is still worthwhile);
- breast pain, with no obvious discrete lumps in the breast, and no benefit from routine treatments.

Although the guidelines say that there is no need for your family doctor to arrange any tests, since these will all be done at the breast clinic, they should be able to answer any questions that you are worried about, and offer advice on how to get more information about breast cancer if you want it.

6

Breast clinics and
multi-disciplinary teams

The breast clinic

Over the last ten years breast clinics at hospitals have become
very efficient and streamlined. This means that you shouldn't have
to wait long for an appointment, and when you do attend the clinic
everything will be done to give you answers as quickly as
possible. Most breast clinics run a 'one-stop' 'triple-assessment'
system: this means that in a single visit you will see a specialist
breast surgeon who will talk to you and then examine you.
Sometimes, if a lump is very obviously non-cancerous, this is all
that is needed, but if there is the slightest doubt about the
diagnosis then they will arrange a mammogram (often with an
ultrasound examination, which is done at the same time), and if
necessary use a needle to take a small sample of tissue from the
breast lump (a biopsy). This sample can be looked at under the
microscope to see whether or not there is a cancer present. Very
often you will get an answer while you are at the clinic, on the
same day or within a couple of days afterwards. The whole system
is designed to try and tell you what is wrong, and whether or not
you have cancer, as quickly as possible, so that the worry and
anxiety of waiting for news is kept to a minimum. If the news is
that you do have cancer then the aim is to break that news as
sympathetically and reassuringly as possible, giving you a clear
idea of what can be offered in the way of treatment and the likely
outcome of that treatment. So you know not only what is wrong
but also what will happen next, and have some idea of what the
future might hold.

Who's who in breast cancer care

This is probably a good place to introduce the people who will
make up the team which will look after you if the tests confirm

33

that you have breast cancer. Some of them you will meet face to face and others will be working behind the scenes.

The breast surgeon

It is estimated that in most hospitals breast surgery (which includes benign conditions as well as cancer) makes up about a quarter of the surgical workload. This means that nowadays there are surgeons who specialize in diseases of the breast and do little other work besides. This contrasts with ten or twenty years ago, when breast surgery was part of the role of general surgeons who did a wide range of other operations. Your breast surgeon will be an expert, and will have specialist knowledge and experience in the treatment of breast cancer. He or she will usually be the first hospital consultant you will see, and will be responsible for making the diagnosis and carrying out the first-line treatment of your cancer.

The breast-care nurse

All breast clinics have specialist breast-care nurses, and they will usually be there when the surgeon gives you the news of whether or not you have a cancer. Once the surgeon has told you about how matters stand and outlined the possible treatment, the breast-care nurse will be able to talk to you and start to put in place the support to help you through your cancer journey. Your nurse will understand the shock and distress that the news of your cancer will have caused, and will be experienced in helping you to cope and come to terms with this. He or she will provide another layer of information, advice and guidance to back up what you have been told by your doctors, and will be there to support you throughout the entire time of your treatment and your long-term follow-up afterwards.

The clinical oncologist

An oncologist is a doctor who specializes in cancer treatment. Clinical oncologists used to be called radiotherapists, because they are the doctors who provide radiotherapy, but they are also qualified to give hormone treatments and chemotherapy, so the name of their specialism was changed to clinical oncology to reflect this wider role. If you are going to have radiotherapy then this part of your treatment will be under the care of a clinical oncologist, and they may or may not supervise any chemotherapy or hormone treatment that you might need.

The therapy radiographer

Rather confusingly, these days therapy radiographers are often called radiotherapists. They are the people who will actually deliver your radiotherapy and will see you each time you come to have your treatment.

The medical oncologist

Medical oncologists are cancer specialists who deal only with drug treatment, and don't do any radiotherapy. If you need drug treatment, with hormones or chemotherapy, then you may be referred to a medical oncologist for this.

The chemotherapy nurses

Although a consultant clinical or medical oncologist will be in charge of your drug treatment, any chemotherapy that you have will actually be given by specialist chemotherapy nurses, and they will also do a lot of the routine check-ups during the time you are having your chemotherapy.

The radiologist

This is the doctor who will arrange any X-rays or scans that you need and will report on those tests, which will help to make the diagnosis, and who will also look at whether or not your cancer has spread.

The pathologist

The pathologist will look at the samples of tissue (biopsies) that are taken from your breast when you first come to the clinic, and confirm whether or not you have a cancer. If you go on to have surgery they will examine your cancer, and the lymph glands from under your arm, to find out exactly what type of cancer it is, how big it is, what the grade of the cancer is, whether it has been completely removed or whether there might be traces of cancer still in your breast, and whether or not it has spread to the lymph nodes under your arm. All these things are very important in working out whether or not you need any further treatment after your surgery.

Multi-disciplinary teams

When you first go to the breast clinic you will probably meet only your surgeon and specialist breast-care nurse. But once the diagnosis has been made and you have had your initial operation to remove the cancer, then the various experts will get together to decide whether or not you need any further treatment, and to work out what that treatment should be. They do this at regular multi-disciplinary team meetings, and everyone who has a breast cancer diagnosed will be discussed at these meetings. This means that although you may see only one specialist at any one time, the treatments that they recommend to you will be the result of thought and discussion by a panel of experts, so that you get the best possible advice.

Depending on the decisions of the multi-disciplinary team, you may not need any further treatment, in which case your breast surgeon will continue to keep an eye on you, or they may recommend that you see either the consultant clinical or medical oncologist to talk about what else may be necessary.

7
Surgery

For many women, one of the major fears that still surround the discovery of a breast cancer is the prospect of surgery. Some form of operation will almost always be needed to remove the tumour.

For many years of the last century a radical mastectomy was the commonest type of surgery for breast cancer. This was a big operation, taking away not only the breast but also the muscles behind it, leaving just a thin covering of skin over the ribs. It was a very disfiguring operation, and was usually followed by a course of high-dose old-fashioned radiotherapy which could lead to further skin damage and scarring. Happily, these days the situation is very different.

The choice of operations lies between a mastectomy and a breast-sparing, or conservative, approach.

Mastectomy

A mastectomy will mean taking away the breast, the skin covering the breast and the nipple, but it is only very rarely that surgeons feel it is necessary to remove the underlying muscle. This operation, known as a simple mastectomy, leaves a good covering of tissue on the chest so, apart from the disappearance of the breast, there is no disfigurement, just a smooth covering of skin over the chest with a scar from the surgery. The scar is usually no more than a single fine line running across the chest, which gradually fades to become almost unnoticeable.

Nowadays two alternative types of mastectomy may be possible for very early cancers, or when the mastectomy is done as a way of preventing breast cancer in women who are at very high risk of getting the disease. These are called a skin-sparing mastectomy and a subcutaneous mastectomy. In a skin-sparing mastectomy, the surgeon makes one or more small cuts in the skin of the breast, usually around the nipple, and takes away the nipple and the areola (the pigmented circle of skin around the nipple) and underlying breast tissue through these incisions but is able to leave behind the original skin of the rest of the breast. In a subcutaneous mastectomy the surgeon usually makes a cut in the skin fold under the breast (the infra-mammary fold) and through this takes away all the breast tissue, but leaves behind the skin of the breast with the nipple and areola intact. After either of these procedures the shape of the breast can be restored by some form of breast reconstruction (see p. 41).

Conservative breast surgery

When it comes to conservative surgery several different operations are possible, but they all involve taking away the cancer with a margin of normal tissue around it. For most tumours a lumpectomy (also known as a wide local excision) is the usual approach, removing the lump of cancer with a collar of about a centimetre of normal tissue around it. The change in the appearance of the breast after surgery will depend on both the size of the breast and the size of the cancer. A small cancer removed from a large breast will make little or no difference to the shape of that breast, whereas a larger cancer removed from a small breast will make quite a big difference to its appearance.

Sometimes a slightly bigger operation is done, taking away about a quarter of the breast tissue. This called a quadrantectomy, or segmental resection. This will lead to a more obvious change in the shape of the breast, especially for women who have smaller breasts.

Making your choice

Occasionally a surgeon will advise that a mastectomy is essential to give the best chance of a cure, but usually the choice of operation is very much your decision.

Things that may make a surgeon decide you need a mastectomy include having a large cancer, or having a cancer that lies directly behind the nipple, or having cancer in several different parts of the same breast (this is called a multifocal primary breast cancer).

If the decision on the type of surgery is left in your hands then the appearance of your breast after surgery is likely to be important in making up your mind, and most breast surgeons will be able to show you a selection of 'before and after' photographs to give you an idea of how things might look after different types of surgery. It may even be possible to meet other women who have had breast surgery, and talk to them, and see how they have been affected and what they thought of the results.

A word about radiotherapy

Just as things have improved in surgery, so they have in radiotherapy. The severe skin damage that was seen with treatment thirty or forty years ago is long gone. Today there may well be some temporary redness and soreness of the skin, like a mild sunburn, for a week or two after the end of treatment, but this will rapidly settle and the skin will go back to its normal appearance. Over the years after radiotherapy, however, the breast may shrink in size a little and become slightly smaller, although this usually is not very obvious. Because some fibrous tissue forms in the breast after radiotherapy it may also become a little bit firmer to the touch, and feel a little bit more solid than your other breast, but once again this is usually a slight change and not very obvious.

Surgery to the axilla

Whatever type of breast operation you choose, your surgery will always include a look at the tissues of the armpit, the axilla, on that side of your body. This is because it is very important to know whether or not your cancer has spread into the lymph glands under your arm, and the only way this can be done is to take some of those glands away so that they can be looked at under the microscope.

The two types of operation that have usually been done are

lymph node sampling, where some of the glands are taken away for examination, and lymph node clearance (axillary clearance), where the surgeon tries to remove all the lymph nodes in that area. Your surgeon should discuss with you the benefits and risks of these two different types of operation, and give you advice as to which might be better in your case. More recently, another approach is something called sentinel node biopsy; this is discussed in more detail in Chapter 9, and you might like to ask your surgeon about this.

Breast prostheses

An important part of modern-day breast surgery is thinking about the cosmetic appearance of your breast after surgery. There are two main approaches to this: the use of breast prostheses (false breasts), and breast reconstruction. Restoring the shape of the breast and make everything look as normal as possible is most often a problem for women having a mastectomy, but if a more conservative operation has made a big change to the appearance of the breast then this too might need attention.

Prostheses (false breasts) are most often used after a mastectomy but are sometimes offered to women who have had a lumpectomy or wide local excision if this has noticeably altered the shape of their breast. There are a number of different types of breast prosthesis. For the first month or so after surgery the tissues will still be tender and healing, and at this stage you are likely to be given a lightweight soft foam prosthesis (this is sometimes called a cumfie or softie) which you can put inside your bra.

When everything is fully healed you will be fitted with a permanent prosthesis. This is most often made from silicone, and has a similar feel to normal breast tissue. In the past there have been some doubts about the safety of silicone prostheses but they are now considered absolutely safe to use. The prosthesis is designed to sit inside your bra and to reproduce as closely as possible the shape of your previous breast. Some prostheses also reproduce the shape of a nipple on their surface.

Although silicone prostheses are similar in weight to normal breast tissue, some women do find them rather heavy, and if this is a problem for you then lighter types of prosthesis are available. The fitting of your breast prosthesis will usually be arranged by your breast-care nurse. The fitting service, and the prosthesis, is free of charge on the NHS. If you prefer, Breast Cancer Care also offers a free fitting service (address on p. 105) but you may have to travel to get this. The prostheses are replaced every two years, or sooner if they become unduly worn or damaged; again, this is free of charge.

Breast reconstruction

If you are going to have a mastectomy then your surgeon should discuss the possibility of breast reconstruction with you; if they don't, and if this is something you think you might want, then you should certainly ask about it.

A breast reconstruction may be done at the time of your initial operation to remove the cancer – this is called an immediate reconstruction – or it may take place some weeks or months later – this is called a delayed reconstruction. There are also a number of different types of breast reconstruction surgery. So if you are thinking about a reconstruction, your surgeon will want to discuss both the timing and the type of operation with you.

The surgery for breast reconstruction will often be done by a specialist plastic surgeon, rather than your breast surgeon. Sometimes breast and plastic surgeons work together in joint clinics, so you may be able to see them at the same time, but often it will mean that you will need a separate appointment, sometimes with a visit to a different hospital, in order to meet your plastic surgeon and discuss the details of what might be on offer in your case.

Once a breast cancer has been discovered it is important to remove it as quickly as possible. Not all breast clinics are able to offer immediate reconstruction because of local waiting lists for the operation. Also, if you are going to have radiotherapy, surgeons will often recommend that reconstruction is delayed until that treatment is completed, since the radiation can sometimes affect the appearance of the new breast.

Types of breast reconstruction

There are a number of different types of breast reconstruction. These fall into two main groups, using either an implant or your own tissue to build up the new breast shape. With an implant, the surgeon will usually make a pocket under the skin on the chest and slip in either a silicone gel implant of the right size to make good the defect or an expandable implant which can be gradually inflated over a period of weeks or months by injecting salt solution (saline) into it until it reaches the correct size and shape. Although the initial operation will have to be done as an inpatient, the injections to inflate the implant are done as an outpatient, taking only a few minutes, and cause little or no discomfort.

Breast reconstruction using your own tissue to make the new breast involves more complicated surgery and may mean several operations, with more scars, but some women feel that the end result is a more natural-feeling breast and prefer this approach. This is one of those situations where everyone is different, and you will have quite a lengthy chat with your surgeon to go through all the different options, with time to decide which is likely to be best for you personally.

It is also true to say that many women who at first feel they would like to have a reconstruction find after a few months, when they have fully recovered from surgery and adjusted to their new appearance, that actually they are quite happy to stay as they are. Another thing to remember is that although the surgeons are very skilful they can never give you a new breast that is exactly the same as before your original operation; it will always look and feel different.

Nipple reconstruction

Reconstruction with either an implant or your own tissues can help restore something of the shape and feel of the breast but does not reproduce your nipple; if you want this then there are several choices available, but they do mean some further surgery.

If your surgeon is sure there is no risk of any cancer cells in

SURGERY

your nipple area, then it may be possible to preserve your nipple, and the skin immediately around it (the areola), and graft it on to your reconstructed breast. Another option is nipple reconstruction, where a new nipple is formed, either by taking some tissue from the nipple on your other breast (this is called nipple sharing) or making a new nipple from a small flap of skin on your newly constructed breast. This new skin-coloured nipple can be tattooed, using special creams injected under a local anaesthetic, to give it the correct colour to match your other nipple. If you do not like the idea of yet more surgery then it is possible to get false nipples, made of silicone, which you can stick on your new breast with special adhesive. These nipple prostheses can be either bought ready-made or made to order so that you get just the shape and colour that you want. Although these different approaches can all help restore the appearance of your nipple, unfortunately none of them gives you back the feeling or sensation in that tissue.

8
What happens after surgery?
Adjuvant therapy

One of the reasons why the outlook for women with breast cancer has improved so much in the last twenty or thirty years is the use of other treatments after surgery to increase the chance of a cure.

Although an operation will usually remove all traces of breast cancer, if nothing more is done then some women will find, months or years later, that their cancer has come back. This may be with a recurrence in the breast itself, or the nearby lymph nodes under the arm, or in some other part of the body like the bones, the liver, the lungs or the brain. These islands of tumour spread are called secondary cancers, or metastases.

In fact these secondary cancers will have been present when the initial breast cancer was removed, but at that time they would have been microscopic seedlings of cancer, far too small to show up on any examinations or tests. They would have been completely undetectable. But over time they carry on growing and eventually cause symptoms that lead to their discovery.

So for some women their initial operation, the removal of their breast cancer and some, or all, of the axillary lymph nodes, will bring about a complete cure. But for others, although the operation seems to have been a success, the presence of microscopic, hidden seedlings of cancer that are still present will mean that the condition will come back unless more treatment is given to destroy those seedlings.

The treatments that can be offered to increase the chances of a cure after surgery are radiotherapy, chemotherapy and hormone therapy.

The use of these different therapies to try and reduce the risk of the cancer coming back in women whose cancer appears to have been taken away by surgery is called 'adjuvant therapy'.

44

Radiotherapy

Radiotherapy involves a course of treatment as an out-patient over about three to six weeks. The treatment is focused on the remaining tissue of the affected breast, and the aim of treatment is to prevent any recurrence of the cancer in that breast. Radiotherapy will be recommended to almost all women who have a conservative operation, and some women who have had a mastectomy may also be advised to have radiotherapy after their operation, although this is less common.

Usually the treatment is given on a daily basis, Monday to Friday, with a break at weekends, although the pattern does vary from hospital to hospital. Each treatment involves lying on a couch under a big machine, called a Linear Accelerator. The machine does not touch you but produces a beam of X-rays which are focused on your breast area. The treatment itself is quite painless – you don't feel anything from it, and there are no immediate side-effects (so normally it is quite OK to drive yourself to and from the hospital). Each treatment lasts about 15 to 20 minutes, but most of that time is spent getting you ready and in the right position, and making various checks. The time when you will be in the treatment room on your own, with the machine switched on, is only a matter of a couple of minutes at each visit.

It is important that your treatment is given accurately, to irradiate exactly the right area, and this will mean one or two visits before you start your course of radiotherapy, to have various measurements made and X-rays or scans taken in order to plan the technical side of your radiation.

Chemotherapy

Chemotherapy is also usually given as an out-patient or day-patient, and involves regular visits to hospital over four to eight months. Unlike radiotherapy, which is directed just to the breast area, chemotherapy goes into the bloodstream and spreads to all parts of the body. So it is given if doctors suspect there may be cancer cells that have spread beyond the breast to form microscopic secondary cancers in other places.

The chemotherapy involves giving drugs into your veins. This may be done with a drip connected to a special needle (called a canula), which is put into one of the veins of your arm on the opposite side to where you had your surgery, or you may be offered a central line or a PICC line. These are special tubes which are placed either into a vein just below your collar-bone or in the bend of your elbow; they can stay in place throughout the time of your chemotherapy treatment, and can be used for taking blood tests as well as for actually giving the drugs. So having a line in place avoids the need for lots of pin pricks, and is especially good if you don't like needles.

Hormone therapy

Hormone therapy usually means taking tablets or occasionally, in younger women who haven't reached the menopause, it may mean injections once every few months, which are into the tissues under the skin on the front of the tummy.

Like chemotherapy, hormone treatment affects all parts of the body, and so is used if it is thought that there is a risk that the cancer might have spread. But hormone therapy only works if the cancer has oestrogen receptors – if it is ER+. So only women who have had ER+ cancers will be offered hormone treatment.

Who needs adjuvant treatment?

Because there is no way of detecting whether or not microscopic seedlings of tumour are present, the advice as to whether someone with breast cancer should have adjuvant therapy after their surgery, and what sort of adjuvant therapy they should have, is based on a number of things that are known to increase the risk of the cancer having spread. These include whether or not the lymph nodes under the arm were affected, the size of your original breast cancer (the larger the cancer the greater the chance of spread) and the grade of the cancer (a Grade III cancer is more likely to have spread than a Grade I cancer).

When all the information from your operation is known, this will be discussed by a group of experts. This group is known as a multi-disciplinary team, and will include your surgeon, a clinical oncologist (a doctor who specializes in radiotherapy and drug treatment of cancer), a medical oncologist (a doctor who specializes in chemotherapy and hormone therapy) and other specialist doctors and nurses. They will reach a decision on whether you need the further, adjuvant treatment and, if so, exactly what treatment should be recommended to you.

Some women may not need any further treatment, most will be advised to have radiotherapy, and some will be offered either hormone therapy or chemotherapy, or both, as well. Incidentally, if you are having hormone therapy and chemotherapy it is usual not to give them at the same time, and you will be advised to stop any hormone tablets or injections that you are having while you have your course of chemotherapy, and restart them once your chemotherapy is completed. This is because the hormone treatment can make chemotherapy less effective if it is given at the same time.

Side-effects of treatment

The main worry that people have about radiotherapy, chemotherapy and hormone therapy is over the possible side-effects of treatment. The likelihood of side-effects, the sort of things you might experience and how troublesome they might be, varies very much with the three different types of treatment.

Radiotherapy

With radiotherapy the main side-effects are tiredness and soreness. About half of those who have a course of radiotherapy for breast cancer will find that they feel very tired after their first few treatments, and this tiredness will last throughout their course of radiation. Once the radiotherapy has ended then that tiredness will usually disappear over a period of a few weeks to a couple of months. Why some people feel really worn out by radiotherapy while others, having exactly the same treatment, feel no tiredness at all remains a mystery.

Most women having radiotherapy will notice some slight pinkness and soreness of the skin and remaining breast tissue towards the end of their course of radiotherapy. For a few women this may become really uncomfortable, with reddening and even very occasionally some blistering of the skin. The radiotherapists who are giving you your treatment will be able to offer creams and lotions to help this, and the changes are very temporary. Usually within four to six weeks of finishing radiotherapy things will be more or less back to normal. Once again, why some women get a lot of soreness and discomfort during, and for a week or two after, their radiation while others get virtually no upset is a puzzle, although, as a general rule, women with larger breasts are more likely to have problems with soreness.

There are also some longer-term changes that might occur months after radiotherapy to the breast. The commonest of these is some shrinkage of the breast tissue, which takes place gradually over a period of a couple of years after treatment. If this does happen the change is generally quite a small one, but sometimes the reduction in the size of the breast may be more obvious. Occasionally this shrinkage is accompanied by some thickening of the breast tissue (called fibrosis) which can make your breast feel much firmer than before. The radiotherapy does also lead to some thinning of the bones where the treatment is given, so your ribs may become a bit more brittle, and this can increase the risk of fractures if you have a fall or an injury. In the past radiotherapy could lead to some late damage to the heart muscle and the lungs, but with improvements over the last twenty years in the way treatment is given these side-effects are now very rare indeed.

Chemotherapy

The side-effects of chemotherapy depend on the drugs that are used and the doses that are given. A wide range of different chemotherapy drugs can be used against breast cancer, and the side-effects of the drugs which are used do vary. It is also true to say that individuals differ in their tolerance of treatment: two people may have exactly the same drugs, at exactly the same doses, and one may feel right as rain and the other absolutely dreadful.

The commonest side-effects with chemotherapy are tiredness, sickness, hair loss and a low blood count (which increases your risk of picking up infections). Nearly everyone having chemotherapy will feel a degree of tiredness. For some people this will be a slight weariness, but for others it will be an overwhelming fatigue, where absolutely everything is an effort. And this tiredness can often last for many months after the treatment is over.

Sickness used to be a huge problem with chemotherapy, but nowadays with modern anti-sickness drugs, which are routinely given along with chemotherapy, many people have no problems at all, and for those that do it is usually only a minor nuisance rather than a major distress.

Nearly all chemotherapy drugs have an effect on the blood count, particularly on the white blood cells, which help protect against infection. Usually, although the white cell count falls after a dose of chemotherapy, you don't actually feel any symptoms from this. But you will always get advice about looking out for, and protecting against, infections, and you will have regular blood tests before each dose of chemotherapy to check that your blood count is OK.

Although your doctors will decide what chemotherapy is best for you, and will keep an eye on your progress through treatment, your drugs will be given by specialist chemotherapy nurses, and they will guide and support you through the treatment and help you to cope with any side-effects you experience.

Hormone therapy

Generally hormone therapies cause far fewer, and less trouble-some, side-effects than chemotherapy. Many women have virtu-ally no problems at all from their hormonal treatment. Having said this, for a small minority of women the therapy can be very upsetting. The most common problems are unpleasant menopausal side-effects. These include hot flushes, drenching sweats, vaginal dryness and soreness, mood swings, and irritability, loss of concentration and difficulty in remembering things. A variety of things can be done to try and ease these symptoms, and because this is a very common problem these will be described here in a bit more detail.

Managing menopausal symptoms

For many women having hormone treatment hot flushes can be a

49

big problem. These often occur along with drenching sweats, palpitations and feelings of anxiety or irritability, all of which can be very upsetting. These symptoms all relate to suppression of the ovaries, and there are a number of ways to try and help.

If you are taking tamoxifen then an alteration in the way you take the drug might make a difference, either altering the time of day that you have your tablet, or breaking the tablet in two and taking half in the morning and half at night. Tamoxifen is made by a number of different manufacturers, and although all their products contain the same active drug some women find that changing from one brand of tamoxifen to another does make a difference to their symptoms. If none of these help, then for women who are past their menopause a change from tamoxifen to an aromatase inhibitor, like Arimidex, Femara or Aromasin, might help, and will be every bit as effective as a treatment.

Sometimes simple lifestyle changes make things easier. Taking regular exercise, losing some weight and avoiding getting too hot might help. Also, some women find that certain foods, particularly spicy foods, and certain drinks, particularly alcohol, act as triggers to bring on their flushes, and avoiding these can also reduce the problem.

Many women turn to complementary therapies. There are a number of preparations available from pharmacists and health food shops which contain plant oestrogens (called phyto oestrogens) and may help. The active ingredients include red clover, soy, genistein and black cohosh. There has been a worry that because these compounds are a form of oestrogen they might actually increase the risk of breast cancer coming back, but there is no evidence that this is the case. Vitamin E supplements have also been shown to help in some studies. Although they are quite popular and many women feel they make a difference, scientific studies suggest that neither evening primrose oil nor ginseng reduces the number and severity of hot flushes and sweats.

Another approach is to try either acupuncture or relaxation therapies. Studies have shown that both of these techniques can help some women.

Sometimes prescription drugs may improve the situation. The options here include low doses of the female hormone progesterone, certain types of antidepressants, and a drug called clonidine that alters the blood vessels to reduce flushes and sweats. None of these is an absolutely sure way of improving the problem, but if the symptoms are severe and troublesome they might be worth a try, and it would be a good idea to have a word with your doctors and see what they think.

As the whole problem is the result of treatment bringing on the menopause, it might seem logical to try HRT. Certainly this is often very effective at relieving the symptoms, but its safety is in question: at least one large clinical trial has shown that women who use HRT after a diagnosis of breast cancer have an increased risk of their cancer coming back, so unless symptoms are very severe and all else has failed HRT is really not to be recommended. An alternative might be the drug tibilone, which has some oestrogen-like activity and seems as effective as HRT in easing flushes and sweats. One study has suggested that it might lead to a slight increase in the risk of breast cancer coming back, but a large clinical trial is currently under way to see exactly how useful, and how safe, it is.

Clinical trials

Quite often these days, you may find that as part of your treatment you are offered the chance to take part in a clinical trial. This can often be quite a worrying idea. People imagine that it might mean that your doctors don't know what to do for the best, or that you are just being used as a 'guinea pig' in an experiment. But new treatments for breast cancer, and new ways of using old treatments, are coming along all the time, and these have to be tested and compared with existing treatments to see which is better. If one treatment is obviously better than another then there is no need for a clinical trial, but if two treatments appear to be very similar in their benefits then a careful study is needed to see if one really is any better than the other.

All clinical trials have to be approved by Ethics Committees, which make absolutely sure that the interests of patients are respected and protected. If you are invited to join a trial this will be fully explained to you, and you will be given written information which you will be able to take away and think about before making any decision. Only when you have given your fully informed consent will you actually be entered into the trial. You have every right to refuse the offer of trial entry, and if you do refuse this will not affect your treatment in any way: you will still get the very best care and treatment that your medical team can offer.

9

Some recent developments

Sentinel node biopsy

If a cancer is going to spread outside the breast the first place it goes to is almost always the lymph nodes (also called lymph glands) in the armpit next to that breast. Doctors call the armpit the axilla, so the lymph nodes are known as the axillary nodes. The number of nodes in each axilla varies slightly from person to person but is usually between 20 and 30.

When a surgeon does an operation to take away a breast cancer he or she will also take away some of the axillary lymph nodes on that side to check whether or not the cancer has spread there. They may take a selection of glands – this is called axillary sampling – or they may take all the glands they can find – this is called an axillary clearance.

It is essential to know whether or not the cancer has involved the axillary lymph nodes in order to decide whether any further treatment, like hormone therapy or chemotherapy, is necessary.

Having surgery to remove axillary nodes can cause a number of complications. The armpit is a very sensitive area and it will often be sore for a few weeks after the operation; also, the nerves under the arm may get bruised and this can lead to numbness, tingling, feelings like pins and needles, or actual pain in the arm on that side for a month or so after the operation. Removing the lymph glands can sometimes interfere with the drainage of fluid from the tissues in the arm and this may cause lymphoedema. Lymphoedema is a pooling of lymph fluid which makes the arm and hand swell; often the swelling is only slight but sometimes it can be severe, leading to considerable discomfort and disfigurement. Once it has occurred, although things can be done to help control it, the condition is usually permanent and the arm never goes back to normal. These various complications are more likely after an axillary clearance than axillary sampling, but they may occur after either type of surgery.

In recent years sentinel node biopsy has been developed to try and reduce the risk of complications after axillary node surgery. The idea behind this is the belief that lymph from the breast drains to the glands under the arm along a fixed pathway, always going to a single lymph node, or very small number of nodes, before filtering on to all the other glands in the axilla. The gland which guards this pathway into the axilla is called the sentinel node. So if cancer is going to spread from the breast to the axilla the sentinel node will always be the first to be affected.

This means that the surgeon can do a much smaller operation, simply removing the sentinel node. If that is found to be normal when it is looked at in the pathology laboratory, no further surgery will be needed. If it does show cancer then a further operation can be arranged to clear the remaining axillary nodes. By using this approach many women will be spared an axillary sampling, or axillary clearance, and avoid the risk of complications from those operations.

In order to find the sentinel node, shortly before the operation a small amount of a colourless radioactive tracer and a blue dye will be injected into the breast. These can then be tracked to show where the sentinel node is, so that it can be removed.

The benefit of sentinel node biopsy is that it lessens the risk of complications like lymphoedema and nerve bruising: it doesn't actually increase the chance of a cure. The disadvantages of the procedure are that there is the slight discomfort of having the dyes injected into the breast, and those women whose sentinel node does show tumour will have to have a further operation to remove their remaining axillary nodes. There is also a very small chance that an apparently normal sentinel node may be a 'false-negative', when in fact seedlings of cancer have already spread to other glands deeper in the axilla, and this will be missed.

Incidentally, although the tracer dyes will usually show a single sentinel node, they quite often show two or three glands as 'sentinels', so a sentinel node biopsy may still involve removing more than a single lymph node.

At the present time the use of sentinel biopsy in the UK is variable; some breast surgeons are firmly convinced of its benefits, while others are less certain. A large clinical trial is in progress to

try and provide more information about the true value of this approach, and when those results are published it will help make things clearer. In the meantime, if you are facing breast cancer surgery and are worried about the possible risks from removing axillary nodes, do ask your surgeon about his or her views on sentinel node biopsy and whether or not it might be helpful for you.

Aromatase inhibitors for early breast cancer

About two out of every three breast cancers will have oestrogen receptors in their cells. Cancers which have these receptors are called ER+ (see p. 19). ER+ cancers use the natural female hormone oestrogen to help with their growth. Reducing the supply of oestrogen to the oestrogen receptors in ER+ cancers will usually slow their growth and cause the cancers to shrink. So for ER+ cancers hormonal treatments can be used, which will interfere in one way or another with the supply of oestrogen to the tumour. Breast cancers that do not have oestrogen receptors (ER− cancers) do not usually respond to hormone treatments.

Since the early 1970s the mainstay of hormone treatment for breast cancer has been the drug tamoxifen. More recently a group of drugs called aromatase inhibitors have been developed. The three most important drugs in this group are anastrozole (Arimidex), letrozole (Femara) and exemestane (Aromasin). Unlike tamoxifen these drugs are only effective in women who have passed the menopause; they do not work in younger women.

Since the mid-1970s women with early ER+ breast cancer have routinely been given tamoxifen to try and prevent their cancer coming back after surgery and radiotherapy (some of these women will also have received chemotherapy as well). The drug has usually been given for five years, and then stopped. It has proved very effective and has undoubtedly increased the cure rate for women with early ER+ cancers.

In the last year or two, a number of large clinical trials have suggested that using aromatase inhibitors may be even better than using tamoxifen. These trials have either been direct comparisons of an aromatase inhibitor with tamoxifen, or have compared giving tamoxifen for some years followed by an aromatase inhibitor, with giving tamoxifen alone. Although these results do seem to show a benefit, the improvement is quite small: for every 100 women with ER+ early breast cancer taking tamoxifen, 80 might expect to be cured; if an aromatase inhibitor is used the figure rises to about 83. Other problems are that these trials have not been running that long, and there is no definite proof that cure rates will be improved in the longer term, despite the encouraging early results. Also, using aromatase inhibitors increases the risk of a woman getting osteoporosis, thinning of her bones, compared to using tamoxifen (although this risk can be reduced by giving other treatments).

On the other hand, tamoxifen itself does have side-effects: it increases the risk of getting thrombosis (blood clots), it is more likely to cause unpleasant menopausal symptoms (hot flushes, mood swings, drenching sweats) than aromatase inhibitors, and very occasionally its long-term use can lead to womb cancer.

Once again, the thing to do is to have a chat with your specialist and get their advice as to whether tamoxifen or an aromatase inhibitor would be better for you.

Herceptin (trastuzumab)

Herceptin is a new kind of drug treatment for breast cancer. It is one of a class of drugs known as monoclonal antibodies, and it works by blocking HER2 receptors in the cancer cells, which switches off their growth (see p. 20). Only about one in five breast cancers contain significant amounts of HER2 receptors, and these tumours are called HER2+. Herceptin only works in HER2+ cancers. Herceptin has some activity when used on its own, but it seems to be most effective when it is given in combination with conventional chemotherapy (cytotoxic drugs).

Herceptin has been available for the treatment of advanced breast cancer for some time, but during 2005 several clinical trials suggested that it could improve the chances of cure for women with early breast cancers whose tumours were HER2+. Although these were early results and the long-term benefits remained unclear, they suggested that giving Herceptin with chemotherapy might increase a woman's chance of a cure by as much as 50 per cent compared to giving chemotherapy alone. Understandably the possibility of such a dramatic improvement sparked a huge outcry for the drug to be made available, even though it had not been formally licensed and approved for use in early breast cancer in the UK.

At the time of writing, the process of officially assessing and approving Herceptin is under way, but in the meantime most hospitals are making it available to those women who need it. However, it is important to emphasize that it will only benefit those one in five women with HER2+ cancers. Although it does not have many of the side-effects of normal chemotherapy drugs, Herceptin does carry some risks of its own, not least of which is that it can cause damage to the heart, and the frequency, severity and long-term risks of this problem are still uncertain; this does mean that anyone with a history of heart disease may well be advised to avoid having the drug.

10
Advanced breast cancer: when cancer comes back

Although it is much less common than it used to be, a small number of women will find that when their breast cancer is first discovered it has already spread beyond the lymph nodes under their arm, and reached an advanced stage. More often, however, advanced breast cancer occurs when the disease comes back, months or years after the initial treatment. In either case the treatment is very much the same.

Being told that your breast cancer has come back is devastating news. For many women it is far more difficult to cope with than the first time they were told they had breast cancer. Not only do all the old fears, worries, anxieties and uncertainties return, but there is the darker knowledge that very often the return of the cancer means that a cure is no longer possible. In this chapter we will look at what it actually means when the cancer comes back, what can be done in the way of treatment, how you might feel and how you might cope.

What does it mean?

Breast cancer may come back in several different ways, and these differences are very important because the treatments that might be needed – and the long-term results of those treatments – are also different.

There are three main ways in which your breast cancer might come back.

A new breast cancer
The first of these is with a new breast cancer. Women who have had a breast cancer successfully treated are at slightly greater risk than other women of getting a new breast cancer in their other

breast. Putting it another way, having a cancer in one breast does not mean you cannot get a cancer in your other breast. If you have had a breast cancer, being 'breast aware' and continuing to attend for regular screening mammograms is still important, so that if you should get another cancer you will be able to find it, and get it treated, as soon as possible. In this situation it does not mean that your original cancer has spread to the other breast; the new cancer is just that, a 'new' cancer. Your doctors will probably talk about it as a 'second primary' cancer, and it is important not to confuse this with a 'secondary cancer' which, as we will see, is completely different.

In one way this is not really your cancer 'coming back' at all: it is another breast cancer which has developed, and is not caused by or related to your old cancer.

Local recurrence

The second way the cancer may return is as a local recurrence. This means that either your original primary breast cancer, or seedlings from it, have grown back in the remaining breast tissue on that side (if you had a breast-sparing operation), or in the scar or skin overlying your chest on that side (if you had a mastectomy), or it may mean that the growth has come back in the lymph glands under your arm on the side of your body where you had your first cancer.

This means that the surgery, radiotherapy and any other treatment you had when your cancer was first discovered did not manage to kill off all the cancer cells, and that some of those cells survived and over a period of time have grown to a size where they show up as new lumps. Although your treatment seemed to get rid of everything there must have been tiny, microscopic traces of the cancer left behind (which would not have shown up on any examinations or tests) and which have now appeared.

Secondary cancer

The final way your cancer may come back is as secondary cancer, also known as metastatic spread, or distant recurrence. This means that before your original, primary, breast cancer was discovered, it sent seedlings out into the bloodstream and lymph system which travelled to other parts of the body, like the bones, the liver, the lungs or the brain. Once again these seedlings would have been too small to be picked up by your doctors at the time you were first treated. Somehow, some of those seedlings have survived all the treatment you were given at that time, and have now appeared as secondary cancers, or metastases, in those other organs.

Although these secondary cancers may be in organs like the liver or the lungs, it does not mean that they are liver or lung cancers: they are islands of breast cancer which have spread into those organs, and they behave like breast cancer and respond to the same treatments as breast cancer. So, for example, a secondary breast cancer in the bone is completely different from a primary bone cancer, and needs completely different treatment.

When secondary breast cancer appears, tests will often show multiple metastases, with a number of seedlings in various parts of the body. Understandably this can seem very alarming, but usually only a small number of these seedlings will actually cause any symptoms or problems, and most will remain silent and trouble-free. Also, the number of seedlings that are present does not necessarily influence the outlook; what really matters is how sensitive they are to the treatments that are given. Having one or two secondaries that are completely untouched by treatment is going to be worse than having twenty or thirty that are very responsive to therapy. Incidentally, usually (but not always) secondaries will show a similar sensitivity to treatment, so if one secondary shrinks in size, most of the others will.

What can you do to stop it coming back?

When you first have breast cancer, the treatment that you are given will be aimed at getting rid of the primary cancer, but it will also be planned to try and prevent the cancer coming back. That is why, although an operation may have taken your cancer away, you may be offered other treatments, like radiotherapy, hormones or chemotherapy, to reduce the risk of further problems. However much treatment is given, however many different drugs or therapies are used, there is nothing that will guarantee that the cancer won't come back; there is always a chance that some of the cancer cells may be resistant to even the most aggressive of treatments, and that as a result the cancer will eventually reappear. Happily, with improving treatment, the number of women who are being completely cured is increasing all the time, and the number of recurrences is reducing.

Apart from having the treatment your doctors recommend, is there anything that you can do yourself to improve your chances of a cure? Taking regular exercise does seem to help. This doesn't have to be a strenuous workout in the gym; just taking a steady walk for half an hour a day, three or four times a week, is enough to make a difference. Keeping an eye on your weight is another good idea: becoming overweight does increase the risk of further problems (and is not good for your general health). Avoiding medicines that contain oestrogen is also usually advisable, so long-term use of HRT (for more than a few months) is best avoided if possible.

There is an awful lot written about the importance of what you eat in preventing cancer coming back, but in truth there is really no evidence that this makes any difference at all. So eat what you like (although, from the point of view of your general health, plenty of fresh fruit and vegetables will do you good), but keep a watch on your weight. Similarly there is no proof that using complementary or alternative therapies improves your chance of a cure, although many people believe it does.

How is it treated?

The treatment you will need depends on how your cancer has come back.

A new breast cancer

If you have developed a new breast cancer, a second primary in your other breast, then this is treated just like any other new breast cancer. The first-line treatment will be surgery. Depending on the size and position of the cancer in your breast, and your own wishes, this may be either a mastectomy or a breast-sparing operation, like a lumpectomy, followed by a course of radiotherapy. The size and grade of your new cancer, whether or not it has spread to the lymph nodes under your arm, and whether or not it is ER+ or HER2+ will decide what further treatment may or may not be necessary, like hormone tablets or chemotherapy. In other words, the treatment for your new breast cancer will probably be very similar to the treatment that you had first time round.

Local recurrence

If you have a local recurrence, then, if possible, the first-line approach to treatment will usually be surgery. If you had a conservative, breast-sparing operation to begin with and the cancer has come back within your remaining breast tissue, then the most likely approach will be to have a mastectomy to take everything away. Similarly, if the cancer has come back in the glands under your arm, then an axillary clearance, an operation to take away all the lymph glands under your arm, is likely to be recommended.

Depending on whether your cancer is ER+ or ER–, or has HER2 receptors or not, further treatment with hormones or chemotherapy might be advised. If seedlings of cancer have come back in your skin after a mastectomy, your surgeon may try and remove those seedlings, and then, if you have not had it before, you would be offered a course of radiotherapy to that area. If you have had radiotherapy in the past, then treatment with hormones or chemotherapy would probably be recommended. If you do have radiotherapy, your doctors might still feel that having hormones or chemotherapy as well might be a wise precaution.

Secondary cancer

If you have secondary spread of your cancer, surgery is usually out of the question and will not be helpful. It is very unusual to get a single secondary cancer from a breast cancer: usually there will be a number of secondary cancers, which may all be in one organ or may affect several different parts of your body. Even if tests only show the cancer has spread to one organ, the likelihood is that microscopically there will be tiny traces of cancer in other places as well. Because of this the main approach to treatment for distant secondary spread is some form of drug treatment, which can get into your bloodstream and travel to all parts of the body, reaching cancer cells wherever they may be. Depending on whether or not your cancer has hormone (oestrogen) receptors or not, and on what treatment you have had before, you may be offered either hormone therapy or some form of chemotherapy.

If you have had hormone therapy or chemotherapy in the past, then you can have it again. There are several different types of hormone treatment and many different types of chemotherapy, and if you have had one type of treatment before you can still have one of the other types, which may be very effective in helping things for you.

What will happen?

A new breast cancer

If you develop a second primary, a new breast cancer in your other breast, then the outlook depends on the stage of that cancer, just as it did when you had your first breast cancer. Because you are likely to be more 'breast aware' and notice any change in your breast very quickly, and because you will be having regular check-ups at hospital, second primaries will usually be found before they have had a chance to spread, and so the outlook will be very good with a high chance of cure. Just because you have had a breast cancer in the past doesn't make the new breast cancer any worse: it is a 'new' cancer, and having had the condition before does not affect your chance of successful treatment and a complete recovery.

Local recurrence

If you have a local recurrence, with seedlings of your old cancer reappearing in your breast or lymph glands, then the chances of cure are more difficult to predict. Sometimes the local recurrence will be just that, a patch of cancer that has re-grown from a tiny clump of cells that were left behind after your first round of treatment. If this is the case then there is still a good chance that a cure will be possible.

Very often, however, the local recurrence is the first sign of a wider problem: in other parts of your body there are probably other seedlings of the cancer, secondary cancers which simply haven't grown big enough to be apparent or cause any problems, but which are definitely there and will show themselves at some time in the future. If this is the case, if there are other secondary cancers – metastases – present, even though they are too small to cause any symptoms or to show up when you are examined or have scans or X-rays, then the outlook changes: the chances of a complete permanent cure become very small, although it may be many months, or sometimes even years, before those hidden secondary cancers become apparent.

This is a situation where the prognosis, the likelihood of a cure, varies very considerably from person to person, and you really do need to talk to your doctors to get their view of what the outlook is for you.

Secondary cancer

If you have breast cancer that comes back as secondary cancer, with metastases in other parts of the body, then this is rarely, if ever, curable. This is a painful reality: the fact that whatever treatment you have will not get rid of your cancer. The consolation, the one bit of good news in this situation, is that with improvements in treatment over the last ten or twenty years many women will not only survive but will lead almost normal lives, with very few problems, for some years after their secondary cancer has been discovered.

If your breast cancer is sensitive to hormone treatment, if it is ER+, then there are a number of different drugs that can be given and each of these might lead to an improvement, a remission, with a shrinkage of the cancers, an improvement in the symptoms, for a period of time. And that time may last anywhere from a few months to a few years. Sometimes during this time all traces of the cancer will disappear for a while: a complete remission. Then when the cancer finally begins to reappear your doctors can switch your treatment to the next available hormone drug, and there will be a good chance of another remission, another period when the cancer is controlled and your life can go on relatively normally.

If your cancer is not hormone-sensitive, if it is ER–, or if you have reached the time when hormone treatments are no longer working, then you can have chemotherapy. There are many different chemotherapy drugs that are effective in advanced breast cancer, and the number is increasing all the time. Entirely new types of drugs, like the monoclonal antibody Herceptin, are giving more options for what is on offer. Like the hormone treatments, different drugs and combinations of drugs can be given over a period of time to bring about a series of remissions and improvements, and, once again, each of these can last from a few months to several years.

With all these different treatment options available and the range of useful hormone and chemotherapy drugs, when some people first discover they have secondary breast cancer they wonder if their outlook wouldn't be better if they had everything all together – a cocktail of hormones and chemotherapy to blast their cancer. But clinical trials have shown that using the different treatments in sequence, getting everything you can from one and then moving to the next, leads to better control of your cancer and a longer life-expectancy (it also causes fewer side-effects, which is a bonus).

Just a word about 'words'. When breast cancer spreads to form metastases in other parts of the body, this is known as advanced breast cancer. Many people think of this as 'terminal' breast cancer, but this is wrong. Although the condition is almost always incurable, many women will, as we have said, survive for years after the diagnosis has been made. And much of this time they will be in good health. If the cancer is in remission with hormones, this often means the only impact on day-to-day life (apart, of course, from the background knowledge that the cancer is still there) is having to take a tablet once or twice a day.

Similarly with chemotherapy: although there will be periods when you are having treatment and have the inconvenience of hospital visits and the upset of side-effects, if that chemotherapy brings about a remission then you may have a period of months, or even a year or two, when you need no treatment at all, and life can go almost back to normal. So although your illness may be incurable it is not terminal. Terminal is the time when no more treatment can be offered to control the cancer, and that time may be many months or years from the day you are first told you have secondary breast cancer.

Coping with breast cancer coming back

The news that your cancer has come back is going to be devastating. Even if you are in the relatively lucky position of having a new primary, with an excellent chance of cure, the thought of having to go through surgery, probable radiotherapy and possible chemotherapy or hormonal treatment, with all their inconvenience and discomfort, and the reawakening of all those old fears and uncertainties is going to be a huge mountain to climb. If you have local recurrence or secondary spread of your cancer, where the outcome and future are far less certain, then the emotional trauma is likely to be even worse.

Feelings of anger, fear, uncertainty, resentment, grief, are all going to mix together in your emotional reactions to the news. There is no easy answer, no simple way to getting through this time. Once your head begins to clear from that first shocking impact of knowing things have gone wrong, then the thing to try and focus on is your future.

Because you have got a future. No one can tell you how long that future may be, whether it will be a few months or many many years, but if you stop to think, none of us knows how long we have left. The youngest and healthiest of us could be killed in an accident tomorrow, or could go on to live for another 70 years. Life is uncertain – and precious. However much we have, the important thing is to make the most of it.

So try and think about the people you love, the things you enjoy, the positives that make life worthwhile for you, and put these at the front of your mind as the reasons for winning your way through and seeing another tomorrow, and countless more after that. It's so easy to say this, and so hard to do it. By all means give in to your feelings, have a good cry, scream and shout, smash a plate, kick the cat (but not too hard!), have a stiff drink – but then try and remember what makes life, your life, worth living, and use that as the first building block to reconstruct your new future.

This is a time when you will almost certainly turn to other people for support and encouragement: partners, relatives, friends, neighbours, your family doctor, your hospital medical team, especially the nurses, counsellors, all may play a part. Who you need, who you feel can help you most, will vary from person to person, but simply talking, finding someone who will listen – even if they don't always fully understand or have answers to your questions – and just sharing your feelings with someone else can be invaluable.

At this time people often turn to thoughts of complementary or alternative therapies. If you have been told that conventional medicine won't be able to cure you, then there is a very understandable temptation to look for other ways to get better. The painful truth is that there are no 'alternative' therapies out there that have ever been shown to cure advanced breast cancer. There have been all sorts of claims, reports of miracle cures, responses that astounded the doctors, and so on, but in reality none of these stand up to examination – they are either well-meaning misunderstandings or downright falsehoods.

Complementary and alternative therapies can play a part, working alongside conventional treatments, to help support you during this incredibly difficult time. They can also have a valuable role in giving you a feeling of some control in a situation where it is easy to feel that you have lost all control of your life. But they are not the complete answer, and it is important not to waste valuable time and, very often, large sums of money on things which will not really affect the outcome, will not make you live any longer.

So if your breast cancer comes back, it is a huge challenge, an emotional and physical mountain to climb, but life will go on – for how long no one can say, but that is true for all of us. The important thing is to make the most of it.

11
Breast cancer in men

Breast cancer is the commonest type of cancer to affect women, but people often don't realize that men can also get breast cancer. The condition is much less common in men – the usual figure that is given is that for every 100 breast cancers in women there will be one in a man, and even this probably exaggerates the numbers – but even so several hundred men in the UK will be found to have a cancer of the breast every year.

There is some evidence that male breast cancer is becoming more common, but the increase in numbers is small and the rate of increase is nothing like as great as the 50 per cent increase in numbers which has been seen with female breast cancer over the last 30 years.

There are many similarities between breast cancer in men and women, but there are also some important differences.

Causes

Around about one in five men who develop breast cancer will have a strong family history of the disease, with several of their close female relatives having had a cancer of their breasts (whereas in men who do not get breast cancer only about one in ten will have a close relative who has had the disease).

Among men with breast cancer who do have a family history of the disease, researchers have looked to see if this is linked to one of the faulty genes which are known to be a cause of some female breast cancers. These two genes are called BRCA1 and BRCA2. BRCA1 has not been found in male breast cancers but the BRCA2 gene can occur, although it is uncommon. The figures vary, but probably about 5 to 10 per cent of men with a breast cancer and a strong family history will have the BRCA2 gene. Men who have cancers linked to the BRCA2 gene often develop their tumours at a younger age.

The links between hormones and breast cancer development are less obvious in male breast cancer, but it is known that men who had abnormalities of their testicles, such as undescended testicles as an adolescent, or infections or severe injuries to their testicles, are at a higher risk than other men of getting a breast cancer. Breast cancer is also more common in men who are infertile, and unable to father children.

Incidentally, figures and statistics are always a problem in male breast cancer: because the condition is so uncommon there are not large numbers of patients, and far fewer studies have been done on the condition.

Apart from those men whose tumours carry the BRCA2 gene, male breast cancer tends to occur in an older age group than in women. The average age at diagnosis for men is around 70, whereas for women the figure is closer to 60.

Screening

Because it is so uncommon there is no routine screening for men to detect early breast cancer. Although mammography, breast X-rays, would detect the cancers, hundreds of thousands of men would have to be screened for every cancer that would be discovered, and this is simply not cost-effective.

Symptoms

Male breast cancer almost always first appears as a lump in the breast, and this is usually behind and very close to the nipple. As with breast cancer in women, the lump is normally painless. In about half of all cases the nipple itself is actually affected by the cancer, leading to distortion of the nipple, which often becomes indrawn, or ulceration, bleeding or discharge from the nipple.

A condition that can easily be confused with male breast cancer is called gynaecomastia. This is firm swelling of the male breast tissue which, like male breast cancers, usually occurs around and deep to the nipple. The swelling can vary in size from a tiny button of tissue to a general enlargement of the breast, making it look just like a female breast. Gynaecomastia is the commonest abnormality to occur in the male breast and has many different causes, but it is always a benign, non-cancerous condition. It can be quite hard to tell the difference between gynaecomastia and a breast cancer just on the appearance or feel of the breast, but simple tests like a mammogram, or a needle biopsy to take away a tiny sample of tissue for analysis, will readily make the diagnosis.

Hormone receptors

Just as in female breast cancer, where the first sign that hormone-based treatments could influence the disease came from work in the late 1800s finding that removing a woman's ovaries (an oophorectomy) might cause shrinkage of her cancer, so in men, some 50 years later, studies in the early 1940s showed an operation to remove the testicles (an orchidectomy), which are the source of the male sex hormones, could cause a remission in advanced breast cancer in men.

We now know that, as with female breast cancers, breast cancers in men may contain oestrogen receptors. In fact, perhaps surprisingly, these receptors are more common in men, with about nine out of ten male breast cancers being ER+, compared to only about six or seven out of ten in women. Also, whereas in women, the older a woman is the more likely it is that her cancer will be ER+, in men age doesn't seem to make a difference: the tumour is very likely to be ER+ at whatever age it is discovered. This means that the great majority of men will have cancers that will respond to hormone treatments.

Pre-invasive breast cancer

About one in ten male breast cancers are still at a pre-invasive stage when first diagnosed, meaning that the cancer is a tumour that is confined to the lining of the ducts of the breast and has not begun to spread into the surrounding breast tissue. These very early breast cancers in men affect only the ducts of the breast (and so are ductal carcinomas in-situ). In contrast to women, men never get lobular carcinomas in-situ because the glands in which these types of breast cancer appear never develop in the male breast.

Making a diagnosis

As in female breast cancer, making the diagnosis is usually straightforward and involves the same 'triple-assessment' of a physical examination of the breast, a mammogram and a biopsy.

Treatment

Once the diagnosis has been made, the first line of treatment is surgery. Because the male breast is so much smaller than the female breast this almost always means a mastectomy, taking all the breast tissue away. At the same time the surgeon will also remove some, or all, of the lymph glands under the arm on the same side of the body.

Because their tumours are almost always ER+, most men will be offered hormone therapy after their surgery to try and reduce the chances of the cancer coming back or spreading. This usually involves taking tamoxifen as a tablet once a day. Originally this used to be given for about two years after surgery, but now it is more likely to be continued for up to five years.

There is quite good evidence that giving tamoxifen to men whose cancers contained oestrogen receptors does increase their chance of a permanent cure, but it is less certain whether giving chemotherapy as well is helpful. This is mainly because of the relatively small number of men who have been treated and the lack of any proper large clinical trials. The limited number of small studies that have been reported would suggest that giving chemotherapy may help, but at the present time most specialists in the UK would probably only recommend it to men who they thought had a high chance of their cancer coming back, and who were particularly at risk. This might include men who had large tumours, or cancers which had spread to involve four or more lymph nodes under the arm.

If the cancer does come back, or if it has already spread to other parts of the body by the time it is first discovered, then once again hormones are the first line of treatment. If it has not been used before then tamoxifen can be given. For men who have had tamoxifen previously a variety of other hormonal treatments can be tried; in the past, benefits have been obtained by giving male hormones (androgens), female hormones (oestrogen or progesterone) or steroids (drugs like prednisolone or dexamethasone). In recent years the aromatase inhibitors (drugs like anastrazole, letrozole and exemestane) have proved very effective in women who have ER+ breast cancer; as yet there is very little information about the use of these agents in male breast cancer, but in theory they ought to be quite effective, and so offer another line of treatment.

For men with advanced breast cancer whose tumours are ER–, or who are no longer benefiting from hormone treatments (whose cancers have become hormone-resistant), then chemotherapy can often bring about a further remission, with shrinkage of the cancer and relief of symptoms. Exactly the same sort of drugs that are used to treat female breast cancer are used to treat men with the condition.

Outlook

It used to be thought that breast cancer carried a worse outlook in men than in women. In fact this probably isn't true. Men tend to get breast cancer later in life than women, and so are more likely to die of other things, like strokes or heart attacks, in the first five years after their diagnosis. Also, there is a tendency for male breast cancers to be discovered at a later, more advanced stage than in women. When allowances are made for these differences in age and stage then the chances of a complete cure seem to be equally good in both sexes.

This means that if a man has cancer which is still confined to the breast or has only spread to the lymph nodes under the arm when it is first diagnosed, his chances of surviving five years or more from the time the tumour is discovered are very good, with a strong possibility of a complete cure. And even for men whose cancer has spread widely through their bodies by the time it is discovered, modern-day treatments usually mean they can look forward to a number of years of good-quality life with little in the way of symptoms from their cancers.

One reason why breast cancer in men tends to be discovered later than in women is a general lack of awareness among men about the condition. Most men probably don't imagine they could get breast cancer. This tends to mean that they often ignore breast lumps – especially as they are usually not painful – imagining that men don't get breast cancer and so there is nothing to worry about. Raising awareness and letting men know that they can get breast cancer is one of the ways to try and improve the results of treatment, catching the disease at an earlier stage when it is more likely to be cured.

This lack of awareness that men can get breast cancer often means that when a man is given the diagnosis he finds it very hard to cope with, not only because of the discovery that he has a cancer – which is worrying enough in itself – but also because of the confused feelings that stem from having a cancer that most people think only affects women. Many men with breast cancer do need a lot of support from their medical team and specialist nurses, and sometimes counsellors, as well as from family and friends, to come to terms with their illness.

12
Coping with breast cancer

In this chapter we will look at some more general ways of helping you to cope with breast cancer. A key point to remember is that these days more than four out of five women who are told they have breast cancer will be cured, and can look forward to a normal lifespan. The news of the diagnosis may be devastating and the weeks or months, or even years, of treatment that may be needed afterwards can often be hard to go through, but in the long term the outlook is good, the future is positive, and focusing on this can be a great help in coping with all the problems along the way. One day life will get back to normal for the great majority of women who have had breast cancer.

The spiritual dimension

For many people, religious faith can give valuable support during the stresses and strains of cancer treatment. This spiritual dimension often provides comfort and reassurance, and gives emotional strength to work through the more difficult days. Prayer and belief can offer hope and meaning when times are bad.

This is a very personal subject, and the beliefs that each of us hold will vary in their nature and in their importance to us. But one general point to make is that, although your faith may be a means of support during your cancer journey, it is not a substitute for proper treatment. Spiritual strength can make living with the effects of your various therapies easier – it may even increase the chances of successful treatment – but it cannot take the place of conventional medicine: the two should always work together.

Talking

Talking can be very helpful. That does not mean it is always easy. If you do want to talk, let people know. Very often family and friends will be worried that asking you about your condition, how you are feeling, how things are going, will upset you, and will often think that by not talking about what is going on they will be doing you a kindness and sparing you distress. So if you want to talk about your treatment, or your cancer, do not hesitate to bring the subject up. Bringing things out into the open will often make for a much more relaxed and easy atmosphere all round among those who are close to you.

Equally, if there are times when you don't want to talk, when you just want a bit of peace, or when going over things again will all be a bit too much, then say so. Let people know when you need some time to yourself, to get your thoughts in order or just to mentally get away from it all for a while. You are in control, so take control and talk as much or as little as you want to.

Talking about your breast cancer and your treatment can have many benefits. Sharing your experience, your concerns, your worries, your problems, can be very positive. That is not to say that other people will always have answers, although sometimes they may, but simply letting people know how you feel can help. It can help because it lets you begin to work out what your concerns are, what things you need to know or do, what questions you need to ask, what support you might need. Just explaining about matters that may be troubling you can often make them less troubling and can sometimes reassure you that your fears are unnecessary, or that something you thought would be a major issue in your case is unlikely to happen or can be handled relatively easily.

Talking also helps you to get a sense of control over your situation. It helps you to sort out what matters to you personally, both positively – things you want to do and achieve – and negatively – things you are worried might happen. You can then decide which of these is important, and begin to plan how to do the things you want to do, and how to find out about, and cope with, the things that are causing you concern.

Bottling things up or keeping concerns to yourself can often make matters worse. When thoughts go round and round in our heads our fears can often get out of proportion, and then the worry just goes on growing. But by sharing your anxieties, bringing worries out into the open, that vicious circle can often be broken, and although the underlying problem may not go away it can be a whole lot easier to live with.

75

There is always the question of who to talk to. A caring and sympathetic partner is the obvious choice – someone who knows you and cares deeply about your well-being, and who, even if they cannot change things, can listen with understanding and appreciate how you are feeling. But not everyone has such a partner, or you may feel that talking in this way is placing too great a burden on him or her – although very often these sorts of conversations can actually deepen the bonds that form a close relationship and bring you even nearer to one another.

But if talking to your nearest and dearest is something you find difficult, then it may be easier to talk to someone on your medical team. The people you are likely to see most of during your treatment are your specialist breast-care nurses and your chemotherapy nurses, and it is likely that you will get to know one or two of them very well during this time. If you ask, they will often be able to find time to chat about your worries with you; once again they may often be able to reassure you that things you are frightened of are unlikely to happen, or give you good advice on how to reduce the risk of them happening or how to cope with them if they do. They will also often be able to reassure you that the feelings you have are very natural ones for someone who is facing up to breast cancer.

Taking this a step further, your nurses may be able to arrange for you to meet and talk to other women who have had breast cancer and had similar treatment, to see how they got on and how they managed the sort of issues you are having to face. In many hospitals this sort of opportunity is offered by breast cancer support groups, where people who have, or have had, breast cancer (and their relatives and carers) can meet on a regular basis and talk together about their experiences. Discovering that other people have had similar thoughts and fears to yours, realizing that the issues you are facing are not something you have to confront alone and can share with others, and sometimes learning from their experience, can often be very comforting.

Some hospital departments also have counsellors available who you can talk to about your breast cancer, your treatment and all the emotional and practical concerns that they are causing.

Although these sorts of exchanges can sometimes be very

valuable, it is important to remember that each of us is a unique individual, and that even when someone has had the same type of cancer as you and has had treatment that may have been nearly the same as yours, their experience of things, the side-effects they might have had, their feelings about everything that was going on, their worries and the solutions they found, may be very different to your own feelings, so do not expect that everything that happened to them will happen to you in the same way.

Diet: what to eat

As already mentioned, there is a huge amount of information and misinformation about diet and breast cancer. Every week stories appear in the newspapers, in magazines and on the television about this or that food which is either good or bad, and there are countless suggestions for diets that will help prevent or fight the disease.

In trying to make sense of all this confusing and often conflicting advice, the first step is to realize that there are two completely separate questions when it comes to the subject of how what you eat and drink relates to breast cancer. The first is: can your diet increase or reduce your risk of getting breast cancer? The second is: once someone has breast cancer, can their diet increase their chances of being cured?

Just two things relating to diet have been shown to increase a woman's chances of getting breast cancer. The first of these is alcohol. Regularly drinking too much does make it more likely that you will get breast cancer. On the other hand, there is equally good evidence that a glass of wine – particularly red wine – every day or so, helps prevent heart disease. So while excessive long-term drinking does increase the risk of getting breast cancer, there is no need to avoid alcohol altogether.

The second thing is your weight. Being overweight, especially if you are past the menopause, does mean you are more likely to get the disease. So if you find you are putting on the pounds, it makes sense to cut back on your food intake and watch what you eat.

Once a breast cancer has actually developed there is no change in diet that has been shown to have any effect on the disease. Despite this, there are countless recommendations given in the media, on websites, at independent non-NHS clinics and by well-meaning people everywhere for diets which will help make the cancer better. Many people believe passionately in these and are convinced of their benefits, but none has been shown scientifically to change how a breast cancer will behave.

There are also many people who claim that particular diets or supplements will help ease side-effects of treatment, and sometimes suggest that they will actually help control the cancer or prevent it coming back. Very often these claims are based on the belief that the change in diet will boost the immune system. Unfortunately there is virtually no evidence for any of these claims. Also, occasionally these diets can be quite extreme, and unpleasant (or expensive), and actually reduce your quality of life rather than enhancing it.

If you do have breast cancer, the two main things that are important about what you eat are that you have what you enjoy, and that you try and keep a healthy balance in your food.

Having a normal balanced range of foods, with plenty of fresh fruit and vegetables, is very hard to beat. For a healthy diet, fresh fruit and vegetables and plenty of fluids are important. Aiming for the Department of Health's recommendation of five portions of fruit or veg every day is a good target, but if you don't feel up to it then don't force yourself. As far as fluid is concerned, try and aim for at least two litres every day. Plenty of water is good to keep the system flushed through, but any other drinks you fancy are OK.

Exercise

We are constantly being told that regular exercise is good for us, and this is true. It is also true that studies have shown that exercise helps reduce the risk of getting breast cancer. Furthermore, there is also evidence that women who have had breast cancer and who exercise regularly have less chance of their cancer coming back than women who do not.

Exercise can also make you feel better. It helps fight off depression, it can improve your appetite and reduce the risk of constipation. It lowers your chances of getting blood clots in your veins (thrombosis) and is a way of taking your mind off things for a while – a distraction from everything else that is going on.

You don't have to do a lot to make a difference. Just taking a steady walk at a pace that suits you, several times a week, is enough. If you want to do more, that's fine, but don't force yourself. Don't push yourself unduly, don't try and take on strenuous new activities because you feel you have to, but equally don't stop everything. If you can manage a short walk, stroll or amble about each day, this will keep your system ticking over and can also provide a period of time when you can get out of the house and have a bit of a change of scene.

Complementary therapies

Complementary therapies are things that can be used alongside conventional treatments like surgery, radiotherapy or chemotherapy to help people cope with their breast cancer. They are not intended to cure the cancer, but are used to ease any side-effects of treatment and improve general well-being.

This is different from alternative therapies, which are unconventional treatments given to try and actually control or cure the cancer. Alternative therapies often come recommended with claimed benefits which sound convincing but have no medical proof; sometimes they have actually been shown to be ineffective, or even harmful, but are still being promoted to unsuspecting members of the public. They frequently involve considerable expense. Sometimes they insist on unpleasant changes in lifestyle, like outlandish diets or coffee enemas! And there are a host of special supplements of 'essential elements', 'vital vitamins' or 'immunity-boosting drugs', none of which have ever been scientifically proven to do any good.

This contrasts with many of the complementary therapies, which are generally used alongside mainstream medical care and which are safe, well understood, can actually be pleasant to have, and usually have a positive effect on how you feel.

79

While health professionals remain completely unconvinced of the claims made by alternative therapies, their attitude to complementary therapies has changed greatly over the last ten years, with more and more doctors and nurses seeing them as useful additions to conventional therapies that can very often improve the quality of life of their patients. Combining conventional and complementary therapy can frequently be a productive partnership.

Many women try complementary therapies to help them cope with the knowledge of their breast cancer, and its treatment. The main types of complementary therapies are the touch therapies (aromatherapy, massage therapy, reflexology and acupuncture), fitness and movement therapies (yoga, Tai Chi and Qigong), psychological therapies (relaxation, meditation, visualization, music therapy) and dietary therapies.

The touch therapies

Aromatherapy involves the use of essential oils. These are plant extracts that have distinctive smells. Each of the different essential oils is believed to have particular physical or psychological effects: for example, lavender and eucalyptus help ease stress, while camomile reduces inflammation. The oils may be used in massage, or given as inhalations or aromatic baths, or applied as creams or lotions.

Reflexology is based on the belief that areas on the feet match different parts of the body, and by applying pressure to these areas energy paths are activated which can produce beneficial effects; so it is a type of foot massage.

Acupuncture is based on ancient Chinese medicine which believes that the body's energy, or chi, moves in pathways, or meridians, beneath the skin, and by inserting needles into these meridians a healing response can be stimulated.

Aromatherapy and reflexology are very relaxing, and many people with cancer say that they feel better after having these treatments. Acupuncture is rather more uncomfortable but there is some evidence that it can help ease pain and sickness if these are a problem. With these different therapies there is at the present time very little scientific evidence for their value, although an increasing number of clinical trials using these treatments are under way, and there is a growing belief that they can be helpful.

The fitness and movement therapies

The fitness and movement therapies involve more active participation rather than just lying back and enjoying the therapy, but many people do find they can help ease anxiety and depression, as well as giving a bit of gentle exercise to keep up overall fitness.

The psychological therapies

The psychological therapies can be as simple as just relaxing in a quiet room listening to restful music, or might involve working with a counsellor who teaches you relaxation techniques or uses visualization (picturing your body and how it is working to fight the cancer or reduce the side-effects of treatment). Art therapy and music therapy, using drawing or painting to channel your emotions, or listening to (and sometimes taking part in) live music performances are other types of psychological therapy. Many people find that these techniques can help ease stress and anxiety and make them feel better during their treatment.

Complementary therapies can have much appeal. They often lead to emotional and spiritual well-being, with a relief of stress and anxiety, and they may actually reduce some of the side-effects of treatment or make them easier to live with. They also offer some empowerment. This is one part of your treatment, and overall care, that you can take control of and decide exactly how and when you want to use it. Furthermore, at a time when, with the diagnosis of breast cancer and all the tests and treatments that follow on from that, it can seem that the running of everyday life has gone completely out of your own hands, having something where you make the decisions can be very valuable.

Each of us is different, and people vary greatly in their responses to complementary therapies. How much they will help in coping with the stresses and strains of living with breast cancer and its treatment varies hugely from one woman to the next – some will feel a real benefit whereas others won't notice any difference.

If you want to try any of these therapies, do check first with your medical team that it is all right for you to do so, and then give it a try. If you find that you enjoy it and feel better for it, that's great; but if it doesn't help then don't worry about stopping. Sometimes, particularly with diets, people start on a new regime and find that they really don't like it but feel they must continue or they will get worse. This is not what complementary therapies are about – they are there to improve your quality of life, not reduce it, and if you do try a new diet, or any other type of complementary therapy, and find that you feel more miserable as a result, give it up immediately.

Times are changing: conventional doctors are becoming more sympathetic towards complementary therapies, and some cancer centres will offer these as part of their service to NHS patients. But unfortunately the availability of these services in hospitals, or at GPs' surgeries, is still very patchy and variable, and the likelihood is that if you do want to pursue any of these options you will have to make your own arrangements and pay for them.

Information

For many women with breast cancer, simply understanding what is going on, what is happening to them, is a very important part of being able to cope. Not knowing what to expect, not understanding what is happening and why, can be very frightening. Your doctors and nurses should keep you fully informed about everything and answer all your questions, but sometimes they don't, and even when they do there may be things you want to know more about.

Information comes in many different forms – the simple chat with your medical team can be very helpful but leaves you with nothing to refer to afterwards. So more and more often nowadays, these conversations are being backed up by leaflets, booklets, video cassettes or DVDs that you can take away and look at afterwards. Then there are books (like this one!) and, of course, the Internet.

There is a vast amount of information out there dealing with every aspect of cancer and its treatment that you could possibly think of. The two problems are getting hold of that information, and knowing whether or not it is reliable.

The Department of Health is very keen for people with cancer to have as much information as they want, so your medical team should welcome any questions you have about where to get this and be able to point you in the right direction. They may offer leaflets or booklets which they have produced themselves, or provide literature from approved organizations like Cancerbackup, Breast Cancer Care, Macmillan Cancer Relief or Cancer Research UK. They can also give you the contact details to reach these organizations' websites where there is a wealth of information. More details are given in the 'Useful addresses' section. You are perfectly free to get in touch with any of these groups yourself and do not need the approval of your doctors first.

Going down this route is probably far safer than a simple Internet search. Although there is limitless good and reliable coverage of all aspects of cancer on the Internet, there is also a huge amount of misinformation, some of which is not only misleading but downright dangerous – just because something is on the Internet does not mean it can be believed, even though it may look and sound very convincing.

Breast cancer support groups

Another source of both support and information can be your local breast cancer support group.

Most hospitals with a specialist breast unit will have a breast cancer support group. Usually these are run by the specialist breast-care nurses. They have no fixed pattern, and so vary very much from place to place. What the various groups do have in common is the opportunity to meet other people who have breast cancer, or who have had it in the past. So you can compare and contrast your views and experiences with theirs, in a social setting. There is often some form of professional input, with informal talks from experts on various aspects of breast cancer, and there is likely to be a supply of suitable background information or someone who can give advice on where to get such information. There may also be other activities, like the availability of some complementary therapies, or access to spiritual support from local faith leaders.

The availability of breast cancer support groups is variable, but if the idea interests you then do ask your doctors and nurses about it, and they should be able to let you know what is on offer in your area.

13

Breast cancer and everyday life

Although it may change, your everyday life does not stop once you find you have breast cancer. Work, driving, holidays, money, sex, friends and neighbours are all parts of day-to-day living that might be affected by your cancer. This chapter is an attempt to explain some of the problems you might meet, and to offer some advice to help you cope with them.

Work and breast cancer

The effect of having breast cancer on someone's working life will depend on the type of treatment they need and their individual reactions to that treatment. For a few people with a very early, ER– cancer removed by a mastectomy, all their treatment may be over in a week or two, while someone with a slightly more advanced cancer, which is ER+, might need surgery followed by chemotherapy and radiotherapy extending over anything up to eight or nine months, and then five years of hormone tablets.

A few people, usually those who have relatively light jobs and understanding employers who allow them to work flexibly, will manage to carry on working during radiotherapy and chemotherapy. But most people find that even if they have few obviously troublesome side-effects during this time, the tiredness that so often goes with the treatments, combined with the need for lots of visits to the hospital, means they have to give up their jobs, at least temporarily.

So if you are working, and find that you have breast cancer, then you need to think ahead about how this will affect your job.

In order to help your planning you will need to know some basic facts about your breast cancer and its treatment. So you should ask your doctors and nurses some of the following questions:

- How long will the treatment go on for?
- What will be involved in terms of the number and frequency of hospital visits?
- What are the likely side-effects, how troublesome might they be, and how long are they going to last?
- What is the likely outcome of the treatment: is the cancer likely to be cured completely?

And, of course, you can get their advice on how easy, or difficult, they feel it might be for you to carry on working during treatment.

Once you have got this information you can start to think about what you personally would like to do with respect to your job. For some people, work is the most important thing in their life and they would do anything possible to avoid having time off. For others, work is a drudge and a chore, and the chance to give it up, even for a while, would be a real bonus. Also, for some people, the diagnosis of breast cancer, and the need for treatment, might give them the opportunity for early retirement or retirement on grounds of ill health, and this may be something else you might want to think about.

When you have got an idea of how you would like to handle your working life during your treatment, the next thing is to talk to your employer about the options available. Most employers will be sympathetic in this situation and try and make arrangements for things like time off, flexible working hours, lighter duties or working from home. If your workplace has an occupational health department or a human resources team, then chatting to them can often give you a good idea of the choices open to you. They will be able to tell you about your company's sickness policies and your entitlements to sick leave and pay during that time. They will also treat their discussions with you in strict confidence.

Employers are usually very supportive of staff who develop breast cancer. But if you do have problems, then you also have rights. Most people with breast cancer will be covered by the Disability Discrimination Act. This Act says that it is unlawful for an employer to discriminate against a person because of their disability. To be classed as 'disabled' under the Act, someone with breast cancer must have symptoms, or side-effects of

86

treatment, that interfere with their day-to-day activities; so if the effects of your treatment will interfere with, or prevent, your ability to work, then you should be covered. The Act also covers people who have recovered from a disability, so if you have been cured as a result of your treatment, your employer cannot discriminate against you because you have had breast cancer in the past.

Under the terms of the Act an employer should make 'reasonable adjustments' to workplaces and working practices to make sure that you are not at any substantial disadvantage compared to your colleagues at work. The phrase 'reasonable adjustments' would usually cover things like time off for hospital visits, changes in your working hours, avoiding physically demanding jobs, or allowing a gradual return to work after a period of sick leave.

If you feel your supervisors or managers are being unreasonable or unhelpful, then you could talk to your occupational health or human resources team at work. If you need advice outside of your workplace then you could talk to your union representative, or contact your local Citizens Advice Bureau. Very occasionally it may even help to get guidance from a lawyer.

Driving

Some soreness and discomfort in the breast area and the axilla is normal after surgery for breast cancer. The bruising of the tissues and nerves in the axilla may also lead to some pain and stiffness in the shoulder and arm on that side of the body. Usually all these problems will settle naturally within a few weeks of the operation.

There are no fixed guidelines on when someone should or shouldn't start to drive again after surgery for breast cancer. So check with your surgeon what he or she feels would be the right time for you. Then, before you actually try driving, just sit in the car and go through the various movements you would have to make for things like reversing, parking, sudden braking and changing gear, making sure that you can do them comfortably and safely. Also check that you are able to wear your seat belt without any discomfort.

A very small minority of people after breast and axillary surgery find that wearing a seat belt is very painful. If this really is a problem for you then you can see your family doctor and ask about getting a Certificate of Exemption from Compulsory Seat Belt Wearing. If your doctor agrees that this would be the right thing for you then they can arrange this, but they are entitled to charge you a fee (although the certificate is free if you are receiving benefits). You would have to have the certificate with you at all times when you were driving, in case you were stopped by the police, but it does not give any details of your medical condition and so does not tell people that you have had breast cancer. But do remember that wearing a seat belt saves countless lives every year in road accidents, and you should only think about applying for an exemption certificate if it really is painful for you.

A final thing to mention is that some insurers have rules about how soon you can drive after an operation, so do just check your car insurance policy to see whether or not this a condition in your case.

Holidays and travel

Usually once you have got over your surgery and, if you needed it, radiotherapy, going on holiday shouldn't present any great problems, even if you are continuing on hormone treatment. If you need chemotherapy, however, this can make things more difficult.

The fact that most chemotherapy treatments are given every few weeks means that it is sometimes possible to go away for a short holiday between courses. If you are thinking of having a short break somewhere in Britain this is usually fairly straightforward, but a holiday abroad may be more difficult.

For a trip in the UK, the first thing to do is to check with your doctors and nurses that they think it will be safe for you to do this, and that it won't interfere with any treatment or tests that you need. Once you have their agreement, then the two things you need to make sure of are that you take with you a good supply of all the medicines you need, or might need, and that you have some written information about your cancer and its treatment. This is a wise precaution, because if you were to be taken ill and had difficulty in getting straight back to your own hospital, then the doctors where you were staying would need to have details about your condition and the drugs you were having so they could take care of you. These days most people having chemotherapy will have their own Handheld Record books giving all the necessary information and contact details, so taking this would be the ideal. If you don't have your own record book, ask your doctor or nurses for a letter that gives all the relevant information to take with you.

Holidays abroad present more problems. Even if your medical team is happy for you to travel overseas, you may have difficulty getting travel insurance. Most insurers will be reluctant to insure people who are having chemotherapy, or who are within a month or so of having completed their treatment. But it is worth shopping around because companies do vary: you may find that you will be able to get cover, although you may have to pay a premium, and they might also want a report from your doctor confirming that it is all right for you to go abroad. Getting insurance is often easier if you are travelling to countries within the EU, or certain other countries with reciprocal health agreements with the UK which mean that any treatment you have there would either be free or relatively cheap. By contrast, it can be more difficult to get insurance for countries where health costs are much higher, like the USA.

If you are going abroad, even if you have got insurance there are a few other things to bear in mind:

- As with UK trips, taking written details of your breast cancer and its treatment is essential.
- Do take a good supply of all the drugs you need (and take some extra in case of delays on your journey). If you have drugs that have to be given by injection, using needles and syringes, or if you are taking narcotic drugs, like morphine, then you may need special permission from the immigration services of the place you are going to, and special documents from your own doctors. Your travel company should be able to advise you, or

89

you could contact the embassy of the country you are hoping to visit.

- Many people with cancer have a higher than normal risk of deep vein thrombosis, and this risk is further increased if you are taking tamoxifen. So if you are going on a long-haul flight, check with your doctors to see whether they feel you are at risk, and what precautions you ought to take.
- If you are hoping to go somewhere where you need vaccinations, this could be a problem if you are having chemotherapy. Because of the reduced immunity caused by chemotherapy, some vaccines might actually be dangerous and others could be ineffective. Once again, have a chat with your doctor if you are going to need vaccinations.

People also wonder about going out in the sun when they are having, or have recently had, radiotherapy or chemotherapy. The skin that has been covered by your radiotherapy treatment will be more sensitive to sunlight and more likely to burn, so you should try and keep this part of your body covered as much as possible. In general, chemotherapy drugs don't increase your risk of sunburn; so as far as the rest of your skin is concerned it is perfectly all right to go out in the sun provided that you are careful and make sure you don't get burnt. Simply take the precautions, with sun creams, sun block, sun hats and so on, that you would normally take if you were going on holiday somewhere in the sun.

Financial help

Sometimes having had breast cancer, and the time you need to recover afterwards, can lead to some financial hardship, and there are a number of state benefits that are on offer to help during this period. They are there for the asking, so do not hesitate to apply if you feel they would help you.

Disability Living Allowance (DLA)

This allowance is for anyone under 65 who needs help with their day-to-day care because of their illness. A special category within this allowance is called 'special rules', and this is for anyone who is unlikely to live longer than six months. A special rules payment means you get the highest rate of payment possible, your claim is given priority, and payment is made immediately. Although the 'special rules' do say they are for people with a life expectancy of six months or less, many people who have an advanced (incurable) breast cancer will find that they are able to get this allowance, even if they live considerably longer than six months. Anyone is entitled to this allowance, regardless of their income or savings, and it is tax free.

Attendance Allowance (AA)

This allowance is similar to the Disability Living Allowance, but is for people of 65 or over. Like the Disability Living Allowance, the Attendance Allowance is not means-tested and is not taxable.

Carer's Allowance (CA)

This is a payment to carers. To qualify you have to be over 16, you must not earn more than £79.00 a week and you cannot claim any other benefits. Also, the person you care for must be receiving Attendance Allowance or Disability Living Allowance Care Component.

Other benefits

Other government benefits which may help include Income Support (if you are aged 18–60 and working fewer than 16 hours a week); Working Tax Credit (if you are on a low income); Pension Credit (if you are over 60 and on a low income); and Child Tax Credit if you have dependent children. Also, if you are already claiming Income Support, you may be able to get help with your mortgage repayments if you need this.

The Direct Payment scheme

Another type of support is the Direct Payment scheme. This gives cash to people who need to employ someone to help with their care. This can include making payments to a close relative, provided that they do not live with you. This scheme is run by your local council Social Services and is separate from the government benefits, which are paid by the Department of Works and Pensions. So even if you have one of the DWP benefits you can still contact your local Social Services department to ask about Direct Payments.

In addition to these various state allowances, the charity Macmillan Cancer Relief gives financial grants to cancer patients who are in need. These can be applied for to cover various living expenses, or for things like a special holiday.

Sex

Sex is a sensitive, and very personal subject. This means it is often something that people feel shy about discussing with their doctors and nurses. Because it is not talked about very much people do often worry, so it is important to start by stating a few facts.

First, no one can catch cancer from someone else by having sex with them. So there is no risk that you could pass on your cancer to your partner by carrying on with your normal love life.

Second, having sex does not make the cancer worse, or, if it has already been treated successfully, increase the risk of it coming back.

Third, having sex won't interfere with your treatment. It won't stop drugs or radiotherapy from working, or make them any less effective or increase the risk of side-effects.

Although there is no medical reason why you should not continue your normal love life during your treatment, many people simply don't feel like it. This may be due to a number of things, including:

- Tiredness: feeling tired, and completely drained of energy, is the commonest of all the side-effects of chemotherapy and most people just don't feel like having sex when they feel worn out.
- Side-effects: chemotherapy may cause other side-effects which are upsetting and just make you feel miserable. No one is likely to enjoy sex if they are feeling nauseated. Similarly, hormone treatments may reduce your sex drive or cause problems like vaginal dryness which make sex unappealing or uncomfortable (see p. 94).
- Anxiety: being worried about your cancer and its treatment is

very understandable, and if you are feeling anxious then you are likely to be less keen on sex.

- Depression: sometimes natural anxiety tips over into clinical depression, feeling generally low and lacking interest in things generally, including love-making.
- Body image: very often, particularly after a mastectomy, women may be very worried about the effect the change in their appearance might have on their partner, and overcoming this anxiety and embarrassment may not be easy. Avoiding sex can be one way of trying to cope with this problem. (See p. 95.)
- The effects of the cancer: if your cancer is still present then the illness itself may be making you feel unwell and switching off your interest.

Any or all of these things may affect your feelings about sex.

The first, and most important, step in handling this change in your feelings is talking. And the most important person to talk to is your partner. Many people find that talking about sex, and in particular their own needs and emotions, is not easy. But letting your partner know what you are experiencing is essential, so that between you the two of you can reach a shared understanding of the way you are feeling. Talking may be hard, but it is far better than hiding your worries and concerns, or trying to pretend that things are normal when they are not.

Usually partners will be understanding, supportive and sympathetic, so once you break the ice of bringing up the subject of sex, finding ways forward together to adapt to your altered desires and emotions should become easier, and you will at least have created a starting point from where you can work together to sort out any problems that your change in sexuality is causing in your relationship.

However, for some couples communication is more difficult, and even just starting to talk together about anything as sensitive as sex may be hard. If this is the case then counselling may be a help. A trained counsellor might well be able to overcome the reservations, inhibitions or anxieties that are holding back an open discussion of the subject, and not only help sort out what the problems are but pave the way to finding solutions to those problems. Quite a few hospitals do have counsellors available for their cancer patients, and there are also sources of help outside the NHS.

Once this background awareness of the situation has been established, you can go on to look at ways of coping with it.

The most likely difficulty is a mismatch in desire, with the person who is having treatment feeling less sexy while their partner's libido remains much the same. This is very natural for both parties, and neither of you should be guilty about the way you are feeling. Once again, talking helps reach an understanding that your physical desires are different, and that that difference is entirely reasonable. From that basis of acceptance of difference you can begin to sort out how to handle the situation. The solutions will be different for different people. They might include an agreed abstinence, a period of celibacy till you both feel the time is right; or you might adjust your relationship to one of hugs, caresses and cuddles showing your love physically without actual sex; or you might change your approach to sex, with a greater emphasis on things like touching, stroking and masturbation, rather than penetrative sex, or changes in position that make actual intercourse more relaxed and less tiring.

These adjustments can only be made by the two of you, and can only be achieved by talking and understanding. There are no rights and wrongs, no set rules, for how the sexual dynamics of a couple should change at these times, so finding out what works for you is the right answer, rather than thinking there is some magic formula that you ought to try and follow.

There are two specific issues which are also worth mentioning.

Vaginal soreness and dryness

Many women will find that they get vaginal soreness and dryness during their hormone treatment or chemotherapy, which can make intercourse uncomfortable or even painful. If vaginal dryness is a problem then there are a number of solutions. There are a variety of lubricants, available at chemists or supermarkets, which you and your partner can use: these include KY Jelly, Senselle, Sylk and Astroglide. Simple glycerine can be used as an alternative, although unlike the others it is not water soluble and so is a bit more sticky. Another alternative is Replens, which again can be bought over the counter. This is a gel which is a longer-acting vaginal moisturizer, and if used three times a week can help to overcome vaginal dryness and irritation.

There are also creams or gels for vaginal use which you can get only on prescription. These contain small amounts of the female hormone oestrogen which nourishes the lining of the vagina and makes it more moist. These include Vagifem, Ovestin, Premarin and Ortho-Gynest. So if vaginal discomfort is a problem do talk to your medical team about it: there may be a very quick and simple solution. Women often worry that using a cream that contains oestrogen may make their breast cancer worse, or make it more likely to come back. In fact, only minute traces of the oestrogen are absorbed from the lining of the vagina into the bloodstream so it is usually perfectly safe, but if you are concerned do check with your oncologist.

Body image

Another physical factor that may influence your sex life is a change in your physical appearance, or body image. The breast is the focus of an enormous amount of sexual feeling, and having any kind of surgery that alters the appearance or feel of the breast can trigger powerful emotions.

Once again, these changes affect everyone differently. Some people take them in their stride and feel that a change in their physical appearance has little or nothing to do with the real 'them', making little or no difference to the person they really are, whereas, at the other extreme, some people feel completely devastated by the change. Similarly, the effect on partners can be very variable, with some feeling that a mere physical change has not altered the person they know and love, while others find the altered appearance more unsettling.

Talking is the key to adjusting to this situation. The likelihood is that if you have concerns, your partner will be able to offer you reassurance that 'you' are still the person they love and care for and that any change in the appearance of your breast, even if surgery has meant the loss of the breast, makes no difference to those feelings.

In terms of physical sexuality, you or your partner might at first find that change off-putting. The probability is that, after talking about it, that feeling would lessen or disappear. But if it remains a tension, then it might be possible to get round it by adjusting the technique of your love-making so that you could hide the change, covering the area or keeping some clothing on during intercourse. Sometimes these new ways of love-making actually lead not only to a renewal of desire but an increase in enjoyment with the novelty of the new approaches to sex.

This section has tended to look at the problems with sexuality. But although there will always be times when sex does not appeal, most people with breast cancer find that they can not only continue to have sex, but carry on enjoying it. And if you feel like it then there is no reason at all why you should not go ahead and have some fun!

Fertility and pregnancy

For younger women with breast cancer, who may still want to have children, there are two particular things to consider: the effect of treatment on their fertility, and whether future pregnancies carry any risk of making it more likely that their cancer will come back.

Breast surgery and radiotherapy will have no effect on the ovaries, and if these are the only treatments you have then your chances of becoming pregnant afterwards will not be affected. The effects of hormone therapy are variable. If drugs like Zoladex are used, these stop your ovaries from working; you cannot become pregnant while you are having them, although once they are stopped your ovaries will return to normal within a few months and having children again becomes possible. With tamoxifen the situation is unpredictable: about one third of younger women who take the drug find that their periods stop, another one third find their periods become irregular, and the remaining third notice no difference. Even for those women whose periods stop completely, pregnancy is still sometimes

96

possible while they are taking tamoxifen (so if you don't want to get pregnant you should take precautions while you are on tamoxifen, even if your periods stop completely). Incidentally, tamoxifen was first developed as a possible treatment for infertility, before its activity against breast cancer was discovered, so the fact that you can become pregnant while taking it is hardly surprising.

The use of aromatase inhibitor drugs, like Arimidex, is not a problem, as these only work in women who have passed the menopause.

Chemotherapy also has a variable effect, depending on which drugs are used, the doses that are given, and your age. Most types of chemotherapy treatment will stop your periods for a time. With some treatments this will be permanent, bringing on an early menopause and making you unable to become pregnant. With others the ovaries will recover after some months, and further pregnancies may be possible. Also, the younger you are when you have your treatment, the more likely it is that your ovaries will work again afterwards. So if fertility is important to you, let your doctors know this when your chemotherapy is first being planned, so that together you can work out the treatment that will not only be effective against your cancer but will also give you the best chance of avoiding permanent suppression of your ovaries.

If you have completed your treatment and your ovaries are still working, is it safe to become pregnant or will this increase the risk of your cancer coming back? This question has been the subject of a lot of research over many years. The overall answer seems to be that it is perfectly safe, and some studies have even suggested that becoming pregnant actually reduces the chances of your cancer coming back and protects against further problems from breast cancer. Despite this evidence, most doctors will suggest that you delay thoughts of further pregnancies for about two years after your breast cancer was first discovered. The reason for this is that if your breast cancer is going to come back that is most likely to happen during those first two years; if you were pregnant at that time it could complicate your treatment, and there might be difficult domestic issues about looking after very young children at this time. If everything is all clear at two years it does not guarantee that you are cured, but the chances of further problems are much less likely.

Friends and neighbours

Having breast cancer can sometimes alter day-to-day relationships with friends and neighbours. Sometimes the changes can be for the better, sometimes for the worse. If there is a problem, then it usually comes down to communication, with either them not understanding your feelings or you not understanding theirs.

Everyone handles breast cancer, and its treatment, differently. You may feel most comfortable by trying to keep things as much to yourself as possible, not sharing your thoughts and feelings with other people, carrying on as near normally as possible. If this is a positive way forward for you, if it helps you feel empowered and in control of your situation and makes you feel stronger, then that is fine. But if you are simply trying to put a brave face on things because you don't want to burden other people, feeling that if you do so you will be letting yourself down or giving in, then think again, because so often sharing your worries and talking things through can be very helpful and supportive. Bringing anxieties and stresses into the open can make them seem far less troubling than bottling them up.

Similarly, friends and neighbours may feel uncertain about how to handle your situation. Should they rush in with offers of help? Should they ask you about how you are getting on, or should they avoid the subject and pretend nothing is happening? They may worry that visiting you will make you tired, or expose you to the risk of minor infections. They may even worry that they could 'catch' cancer from you (which, of course, can never happen).

At the end of the day, it is down to you how you want to handle this situation. If you want to try and carry on as normally as possible, and feel you cope best in that way, then let people know. Equally, if you are happy to talk about what is happening to you, if sharing some or all of what you are going through makes life easier, then again let those around you know that you would welcome their questions and concerns. Or you may just want the

98

practical support they can give: help with the shopping, lifts to and from the hospital, looking after the children once in a while, without the emotional involvement of talking about your thoughts and feelings. But however you want to deal with things, it will make life easier for them – and, more importantly, for you – if you let them know.

Letting them know might be something you find quite straightforward, or you might feel it is difficult and just one more burden to deal with. In this case, getting your partner, or someone close to you in the family, to have a word with friends and neighbours for you could solve the problem.

14
Afterwards

From the first day that you learn you have breast cancer you will probably be longing for the time when your treatment is all over, when surgery, radiotherapy and possibly months of chemotherapy are all behind you and the most you have to cope with may be taking a daily hormone tablet. No more trailing up and down to hospital, searching for somewhere to park, waiting to get tests done and treatment given. Time to yourself, a bit of peace and quiet.

But when it comes, many women find this a surprisingly difficult time to cope with. Suddenly the routine of hospital visits is lost: the regular contact with nurses and other staff whom you have come to know, and who have often become friends who have helped you through all sorts of problems and crises, people whose support you have come to rely on, almost without realizing it. And suddenly they aren't there any more. There is just lots of time and space for you to fill.

All too often that time and space can let worry and anxiety take over: am I really all right, has the cancer been cured, will it come back, how will I know? However well things have gone with your treatment, no one can give you an absolute guarantee that everything is clear. There is, unfortunately, no test, no scan, no set of X-rays that can say for sure whether every last trace of your cancer has gone – only time will tell, and once the hurly-burly of treatment is all over that uncertainty can become a big burden.

That burden may be all the more troublesome because you still don't feel 100 per cent fit. Radiotherapy or chemotherapy may have left you with dragging tiredness that may take some months to disappear completely. If you are taking hormone tablets then these may be giving you some side-effects, which may not be that severe but can still be a nuisance and take the edge off your enjoyment of life.

As with all these things, there is no single magic formula for handling this situation. Each of us is an individual and will cope in

100

our own way. Partners, family and friends can often help, giving you encouragement and taking your mind off things as you find time to get involved in their lives again, sharing their pleasures and problems, taking you out of yourself, and helping to put your worries into the background.

It can help to have something to focus on in those first weeks after treatment is over. For some women this might be a holiday, or a visit to relatives somewhere overseas, or getting ready for Christmas or some family celebration, like a wedding or a big birthday. For others it may be the return to work, and planning to pick up old routines with friends and colleagues at the office, factory, supermarket or wherever.

It may be the time to take stock of your life, rethinking what you are doing and where you are going, deciding what you really want to do. This might lead to giving up your old job, or changing to something new, or finding a different interest in life – going to part-time classes to learn a language, or how to paint in watercolours, or to re-train for some new role. Or it may be the opportunity to do things you have always promised yourself but never found the time, or had the excuse, to do before: taking up golf, spending more time with grandchildren, becoming a volunteer for a local charity.

Perhaps what all these things have in common is that they keep you occupied, giving you a chance to think about something else and not about your cancer. There will still be moments for reflection and – inevitably – anxiety, but you are still very much alive and have a life ahead of you (and none of us knows how long we have got) which is there for you to make the most of. So try and enjoy it.

Check-ups, follow-up

Although the intense routine of treatment will be over you will still need to go to the hospital every so often for a check-up. The idea of this is to see how you are getting on, making sure that there is no sign of your cancer coming back, and asking about, and dealing with, any side-effects you might be getting from ongoing hormone therapy.

The timing of these visits, and who you see, will vary from hospital to hospital. Your check-ups may be done by your surgeon or your oncologist, or both. To begin with they will probably be about every three months, and then after a year or two be extended to every six months. Often after five years they become annual visits, and after ten years are likely to stop completely, since the chance of any further problems at that time is very small indeed. Most of these check-ups will consist of a short consultation, chatting things through with your specialist, followed by an examination of your breasts and the area under your arms, and every so often there will be a mammogram as well, but other tests are only likely to be done if a problem has cropped up that needs further investigation.

But this pattern of appointments is different in different hospitals and is the subject of a lot of debate at the moment. The main reason for this is that surveys have shown that if a breast cancer comes back this is only very occasionally discovered at a routine follow-up visit. Almost always the patient finds something that she is worried about in between consultations, and gets in touch with her GP or specialist breast-care nurse and makes an earlier appointment where things get sorted out. So some doctors argue that there is very little need for routine check-ups, as long as women are warned what to look out for as signs of their cancer coming back and are told that they can get in touch any time that they want to for a routine examination.

The suggestion is that many women would prefer this, as it saves them having to come for regular visits which, even when there is nothing to be concerned over, can cause quite a lot of worry and also some inconvenience. On the other hand, some women find it very reassuring to have regular check-ups where they are told that everything is clear, and would find the thought of reducing the number of visits quite upsetting. So the debate goes on, and it is something that you could discuss with your own doctors to work out the schedule of visits which you feel would work best for you.

How do you know if there is a problem?

How can you tell if your cancer is coming back? What are the warning signs? The most obvious thing is finding a new lump or swelling. This may be in the remaining tissue of the breast where you had your first cancer, or it may be in your other breast. Or it could be in the lymph glands either under your arms or at the lower end of your neck, above your collar-bone (these are called the supraclavicular lymph nodes, because they lie above your collar-bone, or clavicle). Being 'breast aware' and keeping a check on the feel and shape of your breast and the surrounding lymph gland areas is always a good idea, so that if you do think anything has changed or there might be a new lump, you can get it looked at as soon as possible.

When a breast cancer spreads to other places in your body it can cause a wide variety of symptoms. If it goes to the bone it will probably cause pain, most often backache, but any bone may be affected; if it goes to the liver then a loss of appetite, or feeling sick, or losing weight may be troublesome; if it goes to the lungs you might get shortness of breath or a cough; if it goes to your brain then you might get headaches or seizures. But all these various symptoms can be caused by other things, and it can be very easy to be worried that any odd ache or pain, or just feeling off colour, is a sign of cancer.

One way of dealing with this is just common sense. If everyone in the family has had a tummy upset and you develop some sickness, the likelihood is that you've got a tummy bug, and not cancer; similarly if you've fallen over a day or two ago and hurt your back, and now have backache, then the chances are it's due to your fall and not bone secondaries. But if you get a symptom you can't explain, and if that symptom lasts for more than a week and is not getting any better, then it is a good idea to see your GP to get their opinion. Nine times out of ten it will be something straightforward that they can reassure you about, but getting their advice is still a good idea just in case there is a real problem.

A new life

Having had breast cancer is a life-changing experience. Some of that experience will have been traumatic and upsetting, but there will almost certainly be some good things to remember as well. You will in some ways be a different person: you will have faced up to and taken on challenges, handled situations you had never expected to meet and, one way or another, worked your way through them. You are still there, you have survived, and life goes on.

Making sense of it all will take time, but you will have learnt a lot about yourself, and usually the insights that come from this are positive, realizing that you can – that you did – deal with a situation that most people think of as a terrifying ordeal. You are likely to be emotionally stronger, with a justifiable pride in your achievement as a survivor of it all.

Your body may have been battered and drained by the therapies you have gone through, your mind may still be reeling to cope with all the changes in your life. Facing your future may still be difficult. You may feel that the whole experience has enriched your life, or you may feel confused, uncertain or even bitter that fate gave you cancer in the first place. But the fact that you have worked your way through the trauma of being told you have cancer, and then journeyed through weeks, months or years of treatment, with all its demands and downsides, means that you have survived, you have coped.

In fact, when all is said and done, you are really pretty amazing. You can look back with justifiable pride on your progress and take strength from your achievement to build for the future.

Useful addresses

cancerbackup
3 Bath Place
Rivington Street
London EC2A 3JR
Helpline: 0808 800 1234 (for urgent enquiries, 9 am to 8 pm, Mondays to Fridays)
Website: www.cancerbackup.org.uk

A comprehensive information service for patients. It offers a telephone helpline to specially trained cancer nurses, who can give advice on all aspects of breast cancer and its treatment. It also produces nearly 70 booklets and more than 200 factsheets on all aspects of cancer, including breast cancer. There are also more than 1000 questions and answers about cancer on its website (the website also has the texts of all the booklets and factsheets, and links to many other useful organizations).

Benefits Enquiry Line for People with Disabilities
0800 882200
Website: www.dwp.gov.uk
This is a national helpline that gives information about the benefits that are available for people with disabilities (including cancer patients), and their carers.

Breast Cancer Care
Kiln House
210 New King's Road
London SW6 4NZ
Helpline: 0808 800 6000 (9 am to 5 pm, Mondays to Fridays, 9 am to 2 pm, Saturdays)
Website: www.breastcancercare.org.uk

Offers a free national helpline giving confidential advice on all aspects of breast cancer, and has a wealth of publications offering practical advice, most of which are available on their website.

Cancer Research UK
PO Box 123
Lincoln's Inn Fields
London WC2A 3PX
Tel.: 020 7121 6699
Website: www.cancerhelp.org.uk

As well as funding research on cancer, this organization has a website that gives information about different types of cancer and their treatment, as well as a comprehensive list of clinical trials currently in progress.

Citizens Advice Bureaux
Website: www.citizensadvice.org.uk

The Citizens Advice Bureau service offers free, confidential advice on a variety of problems that people with cancer might face, such as difficulties over money, housing or work. The address of your local office will be in the phone book, and is also on the website.

DIPEx
Website: www.dipex.org

The initials stand for 'Database of Individual Patient Experiences'. The website covers a number of different illnesses, but has an extensive section on cancer. This not only gives some background information on various types of cancer, but has lots of stories from people who have had cancer, and gone through chemotherapy.

Macmillan Cancer Relief
89 Albert Embankment
London SE1 7UQ
Tel.: 0808 808 2020
Website: www.macmillan.org.uk

In addition to funding cancer nursing services, this organization provides a number of publications on cancer, including a useful booklet on benefits and financial help for cancer patients (all listed on the website). The website also has useful information on various aspects of cancer, including a directory of local cancer support groups, and patients' stories about cancer.

Index

Most drugs in the UK have two names: a proprietary (brand) name, and a proprietary (brand) name. The first proprietary name is the scientific name of the compound. The proprietary name is the trade name of the drug, which has been patented by the company that makes it. This means that during your treatment you might hear the same drug being talked about but with two different names. With other drugs, where the original manufacturer's patent has expired, often only the non-proprietary name is used. In this index, if a drug has a commonly used brand name it is given in brackets after its non-proprietary name.

Index